S0-BUF-840

THE FOURTH INTERNATIONAL SYMPOSIUM ON MUSIC

Rehabilitation and Human Well-Being

Edited by
Rosalie Rebollo Pratt
August 1-5, 1985
New York City

ML
3920
.I56
1985
West

UNIVERSITY PRESS OF AMERICA

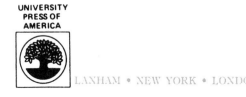

LANHAM • NEW YORK • LONDON

Copyright © 1987 by

University Press of America,® Inc.

4720 Boston Way
Lanham, MD 20706

3 Henrietta Street
London WC2E 8LU England

All rights reserved

Printed in the United States of America

British Cataloging in Publication Information Available

Co-published by arrangement with
Music Education for the Handicapped, Inc.

Library of Congress Cataloging in Publication Data

International Symposium on Music—Rehabilitation and
  Human Well-Being (4th : 1985 : Goldwater Memorial
  Hospital)
    The Fourth International Symposium on Music—
Rehabilitation and Human Well-Being.

    Symposium held at the Goldwater Memorial Hospital,
Roosevelt Island, New York City from 1-5 August 1985.
    Includes bibliographical references.
    1. Music—Physiological effect—Congresses.
2. Music therapy—Congresses.   3. Handicapped—
Education—Music —Congresses.   I. Pratt, Rosalie
Rebollo, 1933-   .   II. Title.   III. Title: 4th
International Symposium on Music—Rehabilitation
and Human Well-Being.
ML3920.I56   1985   615.8'5154   86-28206
ISBN 0-8191-5969-7 (alk. paper)
ISBN 0-8191-5970-0 (pbk. : alk. paper)

All University Press of America books are produced on acid-free
paper which exceeds the minimum standards set by the National
Historical Publication and Records Commission.

The Fourth International Symposium on Music: Rehabilitation and Human Well-Being was held at the Goldwater Memorial Hospital, Roosevelt Island, New York City from 1-5 August 1985. The conference was jointly sponsored by Music Education for the Hnadicapped and the Goldwater Hospital Department of Rehabilitation, Dr. Mathew H. M. Lee, director.

Symposium Committee:

President: Mathew H. M. Lee, M.D.
Vice-President: Meg Peterson
Project Director and Proceedings Editor: Rosalie Rebollo Pratt

Music Education for the Handicapped:

Chairman of the Board: Mathew H. M. Lee, M.D.
Executive Director: Rosalie Rebollo Pratt
Administrative Director: Lynda L. Redd

Music Education for the Handicapped, Inc.
Board of Directors:

Mathew Lee, President
Peter Beach
Dean Burtch
Charles Fowler
Alicia Clair Gibbons
Robert Klotman
Merle Montgomery
Meg Peterson
Donald J. Shetler
Dale Taylor
Frank Wilson

International Advisory Council:

Shirley Harris, Chairperson, Australia
Hunter J. H. Fry, Australia
Frances Wolf, Argentina
John Pauls, Canada
Ole Bentzen, Denmark
Tarek Hassan, Egypt
Daphne Kennard, England
Pamela Smith, England
David Ward, England
Anne Lindeberg, Finland
Jacqueline Verdeau-Paillès, France
Klara Kokas, Hungary
Yoshiko Fukuda, Japan
Kouji Tateno, Japan
Ben Gerits, Netherlands
Jorun S. Mantor, Norway
Graciela Cintra Gomes, Portugal
Alf Gabrielsson, Sweden
Helmut Moog, Federal Republic of Germany
Gertrud Orff, Federal Republic of Germany
Mwesa Mapoma, Zambia

TABLE OF CONTENTS

V. MUSIC AND COMMUNICATIONS HANDICAPS

VI. MUSIC IN INSTITUTIONAL PROGRAMS

Foreword

For those fortunate enough to have attended the Fourth International Symposium on Music: Rehabilitation and Well-Being, the reminder of this historic conference brings back powerful memories about the ways in which music can help the many professionals dedicated to the restoration of human function contribute to the accomplishments and progress of the disabled. The bond between music and medicine is a common one among people and transcends all nations and cultures.

Itzhak Perlman was the honorary chairman of the symposium. The opening day ceremonies began with speeches by Dr. Howard Rusk, the father of rehabilitation medicine, and the late Senator Jacob Javits. Many disabled patients and other individuals sang, played, danced, and recited original poems.

The five-day conference was filled with research presentations, workshops, demonstrations, and exchanges among the faculty and delegates. All these activities helped illustrate the physiologically and psychologically salubrious effects of music when combined with advanced medical technology and music techniques. The expertise of the speakers and audience represented the broadest range and depth of experience in the two professions of music and medicine. The final gala closing ceremony was appropriately held in the Delegates' Dining Room of the United Nations.

A conference such as this would not have been possible without months of planning, obstacles, and even tears. To Meg Peterson, Rosalie Pratt, and Donald Shetler--the MEH trio--my thanks for a beautiful job well done. Thanks are also extended to my Goldwater colleagues, especially Dr. Masayoshi Itoh, for logistical help; and to my family for their moral support and faith. To Rosalie Pratt, our courageous and brilliant music educator, we owe our appreciation for editing selected presentations from the symposium.

This symposium, held within a hospital setting, is unique in that respect alone. It is hoped that this publication will represent current thoughts and trends toward the marriage of music and medicine and will in some way stimulate the establishment of a scientific plane upon which music and medicine may meet, our ultimate goal being the maximum functional restoration of an individual.

Mathew H. M. Lee, M.D., F.A.C.P.
Director, Department of Rehabilitation
Medicine, Goldwater Memorial Hospital

President, Board of Directors
Music Education for the Handicapped

Editor's Preface

The Goldwater symposium marked another solid step toward the renewal of the bond between music and medicine. Music therapy is often seen as an adjunct to psychiatric and psychological therapy. The fact that this fourth MEH symposium was held in one of the world's most important rehabilitation facilities is a great tribute to Dr. Mathew Lee's initiative and foresight, and a clear indication of the direction music therapy and music in special education have taken.

The selected papers of the conference reflect a growing awareness of the resource music can be in the therapy and rehabilitation of human beings. Music is a universal tool available to therapist, educator, psychologist, and physician. The papers in this book describe music and its relationship to human well-being, health care, sensory or physical handicaps, communication handicaps, and institutional programs. It is clear that music has regained the position it was once so clearly accorded by the ancient Greeks.

It is a pity that we cannot somehow capture the very finest moments of the symposium at Goldwater Hospital. There can be no doubt that these occurred during the opening day ceremonies. The memory of the choir of wheelchair patients, the deaf dancers, and the stirring words of Dr. Rusk and Senator Javits is something that will never be forgotten by those fortunate enough to have been in the audience.

This book is another milestone in the work of Music Education for the Handicapped. It also marks the retirement of Meg Peterson as executive director of MEH. Mrs. Peterson's tireless courage, energy, and love for others will always be appreciated by the membership. Her association with MEH will continue as she serves on the board of directors. The officers of the corporation and members of the board extend their thanks and deepest appreciation to Mrs. Peterson. She will always be the heart of MEH.

Rosalie Rebollo Pratt
Brigham Young University

MUSIC EDUCATION FOR THE HANDICAPPED
KEYNOTE ADDRESS

by

FRANK R. WILSON

Mr. Chairman, honored guests, ladies and gentlemen, it is a great privilege and delight for me to be able to join in this meeting that will open--I might say reopen--our eyes to a special realm of the healing arts. This week we will look closely at one of music's longest known and least understood mysteries, its power to foster the revitalization and rehabilitation of the ill and the injured.

The parent organization of the symposium is Music Education for the Handicapped. Its title brings a special need and a special project sharply into focus, beckoning us because of personal and, I would think, intensely felt associations we all make, both with music and with people who bear physical handicaps.

What strikes me about this name, even more than its economy and directness, is its semantic magic. The phrase captures our imagination with three words that are singly as resistant to definition as any in the English language. What is music, after all? What is education? And who are the handicapped? Lest you think I am just indulging in rhetorical posturing, I would ask you to add the word "medicine" to the list and then imagine the adjustments in vocabulary that would naturally take place if just two, or any combination of the many varieties of specialists in musical, educational, and medical professions were discussing the subject of handicaps among themselves. You would not have to get too far along in such a conversation to realize that we only think we speak the same language.

The business of pinning down definitions is not a parlor game, I assure you. The door that now separates music and medicine may be loose on its hinges, but it is still closed. Mutual understanding is the only key that will open it.

I am a newcomer to the world of music therapy. Several years ago, because I had begun to write about the brain and music, I began to hear from music therapists. What they said to me was that no one understood what they were trying to do. I met the President of the National Association of Music Therapists and invited him to appear at the Biology of Music Making Conference in Denver last summer. What I had been hearing before, and what I learned in Denver, convinced me that something must be

1

changed. To an outsider it looks as though a music therapist is a nice person who sings or plays the piano for agitated psychotics so that they will not need to be so heavily tranquilized. To a world hooked on heart transplants and fully prepared to believe in the possibility of brain transplants, the solitary labors and modest goals of the music therapist do not seem to amount to much. I believe this perception to be in error and that you can overcome it.

Should you have a lobbyist in Washington? Should you hire a public relations firm to create an educational campaign about music therapy? I do not think so--at least not quite yet. I think you should take a discerning look at what is happening in the larger worlds of both music and medicine. Change is in the wind, and the future of your work could be very bright indeed.

What sort of change? First, and close to home, there is the simple matter of this symposium itself. It could be profoundly important that we are meeting at Goldwater Memorial Hospital, where New York City's renowned Health and Hospitals Corporation has established one of the largest and most progressive programs for rehabilitation medicine in the world. The decision to bring the symposium here may have been no more than a gesture--you have to accept this as a disconcerting possibility. However, it could indicate a genuine and official interest in the program. If an institution of such stature is actually turning its investigative attention to the healing powers of music, we are entitled to suspect that America's technologic medical industry might be opening the door just a little to some old-fashioned therapeutic sentiments. That would be news.

Now, another event of interest but of equally uncertain meaning. Just across the river, on the *big* island, a program is being developed at a major hospital, not far from a major conservatory of music, to help musicians whose careers are hampered by problems the doctors feel they must try to solve. The same thing is happening in Philadelphia, Chicago, Cleveland, Boston, Denver, and San Francisco. And a short time ago, New York University hosted an international conference to explore the sources and remedies of stress for performing artists. One senses an aura of great excitement in all this activity--a feeling that the musician has gained stature by attracting the attention of a medical specialist who is like the sports doctor. But there are unsettling implications as well; something peculiar must have happened to the professional musical career if it now requires a doctor in the house on a regular basis.

Taking these two nearly concurrent events--a symposium on music therapy and music education, and both hospital- and university-based programs to aid musicians wounded in the line of duty--one is tempted to seek a connection. Whatever your own conclusions might be, there is no denying that a distinct irony graces this coincidence. In absolute earnest, doctors are trying to solve problems that musicians apparently cannot, and musicians are trying to solve problems the doctors apparently cannot.

Permit me to advance a personal theory about this. It seems to me that the worlds of music and medicine are increasingly drawn to one another, when both are thriving and in trouble at the same time.

The problems, such as they are, are evident on both the personal and institutional levels. Advancement and success have become the occasion for an element of paradoxical anxiety and distress for members of both professions. In a few short years, the doctor has gone from handholding on housecalls to a situation that demands the skill and nerve of an air controller at a metropolitan airport; and the administrative, political, business, and legal savvy of its director. The professional musician, in this city at least, faces not a succession of cozy engagements in clubs, salons, or concert halls, but a backbreaking schedule of rehearsals, travel, and acrobatic performances in front of jaded audiences and critics who are not always sweet; and submission to the dictatorial behavior of agents, producers, sound engineers, and the like--that is, when there *is* work.

For those immersed in these careers, there are few opportunities for quiet reflection. However, when that occasional moment does come, it is likely to lead to the nostalgic thought--perhaps fanciful--that things used to be both simpler and better than they are. In music and in medicine, as with other progressive institutions in our modern world, things seem to have gotten out of hand.

At the institutional level, the facts are equally dramatic. Of the many transforming influences in medicine, none is so significant, in my view, as the doctor's raw power to take over the physiologic machinery of the patient. The physician today is a specialist who commands an arsenal of both powerful and dangerous therapies. The patient hopes that these medical intrusions will work but is generally ignorant both of their limitations and their hazards. Whatever resources he might mobilize for his own well being are not often taken seriously. He does what he is told, takes his medicine and gets well, or else.

We all know that this model for medical treatment cannot endure. What you may not realize is that organized medicine, to its credit, is coming to the same realization. A few months ago, I heard Dr. Eugene Robin, Professor of Medicine at Stanford Medical Center, say that the physician's venerable motto, "First, do no harm," really needs to be revised and should now go like this: "At least try to do more good than harm."[1] He thinks it is time doctors look at the dark side of their miracle making--this includes not only the dangers that modern therapy poses for patients, but their tendency to seduce the physician into an attitude of omnipotence. The enormous power granted the physician does not always encourage humility or honest self-appraisal and may cause him to discount the patient's own deeply rooted resources for recovering from illness and injury. Increasingly, physicians raise questions in public about their own power and find the notion of self-healing somewhat less heretical than they did not so long ago.

And what about music? Whatever music may have once been, it has never been the same since Franz Liszt took his magic fingers on the road as a solo act and proclaimed "Le concert, c'est moi!" The idolatry of physicians, if it exists any longer, is far exceeded by the public's passionate worship of the musical virtuoso. Mesmerized by and, to a large extent feeding this appetite, the colleges, universities, and conservatories have been turning out greater and greater numbers of phenomenally talented and skilled performers to satisfy audiences who will pay only to see a high wire act concocted to display the musician rather than the music. The result--our country is flooded with musicians for whom there is no prospect of a successful career.

It is clear that music educators recognize this situation and are taking steps to do something about it. They are developing training programs in non-performance careers, and they are trying diligently to broaden the base of musical understanding and participation among the general public. This will help, but it will take time.

Against the background of these two noble professions now beginning to confront a certain overindulgence in their own success, we can now look at the members of the population whose special needs are the focus of this conference. Swept out of our

---

[1]Eugene Robin, M.D., Professor of Medicine, Stanford University School of Medicine, "Saltem plus boni quam mali efficere conare!" ["At Least Try to Do More Good Than Harm!"], Address to the Permanente Medical Group of Northern California, Berkeley, California, 4 February 1985.

special needs are the focus of this conference. Swept out of our society's manic mainstream, no longer an obvious contender for recognition in a society that dotes on the swiftest, the brightest, the strongest, the prettiest, or the richest, is the individual who is referred to as handicapped. Seemingly deprived of the prospects--might I say freed of the burden--of making the sort of achievement given public notice in our society, this individual is required to enter a labor whose humble object is to regain lost territory.

This happens when the doctor concludes that all that *can* be done medically has been done--the magic show is over. The patient has come through the phase of acute illness or injury alive but left with a physical disability. In some cases the patient is also left with a haunting feeling of failure and learns that the body can no longer be taken for granted. Control of the physical apparatus must be reforged through self-initiative, self-discovery, and self-mastery. The handicapped person enters into this difficult endeavor not to become a commodity, but to reconfirm his or her own physical, emotional, and intellectual integrity. More often than not, he must do this without a great deal of help.

What can the modern physician, or music educator, offer the person in this condition? Where the only treatment left is one resting on the ingenuity and tenacity of the patient, the high-tech doctor pronounces that nothing can be done and distrusts any contrary claim. When the music teacher sees that there are only two concert-worthy pieces that can be played with the left hand, and sees no possibility of a career, the verdict is rendered: "I'm sorry, you have no future as an artist." What can the music therapist offer such a person? That, ladies and gentlemen, is what we are here to learn about.

The music therapist seems to operate under no such restriction, no such handicap of the imagination. As a healer whose medicine recognizes no boundary between body, intellect, and emotion, he or she offers the handicapped person a program in which personal effort can produce change, growth, and recovery of personal dignity. The music therapist also offers this message: a handicap ceases to exist as a physical reality when it has been vanquished as a psychological reality.

I strongly suspect that the formal worlds of music and of medicine are coming close to a rediscovery of their historic bonds. Your contributions could both speed and strengthen this long overdue reunion, especially if music therapy seizes the opportunity to help in the resolution of the serious professional problems in both music and medicine. The process, I suspect, will bring us closer to an appreciation of what those elusive words--music, education, medicine, and handicap--really should mean.

THE REHABILITATION OF THE HANDICAPPED

by

DALE P. DICKIE

The object of rehabilitation is to bring a handicapped person into the community to participate as fully as possible. We are all handicapped, to a certain extent, in some areas of mental or physical ability, but we learn how to cope with minor shortcomings in our makeup. It is the seriously handicapped, however, who need the help of others to reach their aims in life.

Although each seriously handicapped person is unique, we may classify the handicap as either mental or physical. Some are handicapped from birth; others through an accident (the writer adds apoplexy or "stroke" cases to this category); and still others are handicapped by senile dementia, which is reduced mental capacity through advancing age.

How can we help handicapped people? By educating society, by training therapists, and by encouraging the handicapped to try to reach their individual life goals. The educating of society is under way. This can be seen in the many new buildings with wheelchair facilities, in the firms now employing handicapped and mentally retarded workers, and in the literature and films about the integration of less active people into the community. An example of the latter is a book, *So Clear in My Mind*, by Alan Counsell.[1] The book shows the courage and tenacity of a cerebral palsied person in participating as fully as possible in community life.

All aspects of therapy, including physical, occupational, speech, music, art, drama, etc., used alone or in combination, should aim at the most complete rehabilitation possible for the handicapped person. Programs should be devised to suit individual needs under the guidance of the specialists. An example of this might be singing with speech and music specialists, and movement with physiotherapy and music specialists. Additional specialists should be called in where personalized treatment is required. All therapists need to be empathetic to the feelings of the handicapped and, while being realistic about the progress or apparent lack of progress being made at the time, must always endeavor to retain the self-respect of the handicapped person.

---

[1]Alan Counsell, *So Clear in My Mind*, (London: Hutchinson, 1982).

One way to keep the self-respect of the handicapped intact is to offer a sort of "magic" by presenting tasks that have a certain success in order to lessen the very real fear of failure or even ridicule. Until some skill is developed, the goal set should be limited to minimize the possibility of failure. This is crucial to morale.[2]

People handicapped at birth do not need rehabilitation. They need, instead, to learn how to organize and arrange their lives around and, often, because of their handicap.

There are two types of people who need rehabilitation: those who have lived an active life and are suddenly incapacitated through an accident or "stroke;" and those who, because of advanced years, are suffering from dementia or even beginning to withdraw from the day-to-day interests of the world. Music is a major ingredient of success in all rehabilitation programs.

Accident victims (as they often think of themselves) usually had a healthy body before they suffered their disaster. Rehabilitation may occur through therapy. However, the victims often have to relearn skills just as an infant learns controlled movements, e.g., rolling, sitting, crawling, and standing. It takes courage and perseverance on the part of the afflicted and the people working with the afflicted. It takes a tremendous amount of energy from all people involved. Miriam H. Lipman's experience of learning to play the piano after she became blind is but one example of this courage and perseverance.[3]

Singing should be encouraged, for it can relax tense or potentially stressful situations. Singing well-known rhythmic songs relaxes the singing and can often aid the mobility of the handicapped. The writer recalls reading how a lady gained strength and confidence while relearning to walk by singing the melody of "From the Hall of the Mountain King" from Grieg's *Peer Gynt*

---

[2]Dale P. Dickie, "Activities to Put Music in the Lives of the Elderly," New Zealand, 1982. This paper may be obtained from the Education Advisor, New Zealand Council for Recreation and Sport, P.O. Box 5122, Wellington, New Zealand.

[3]Miriam H. Lipman, "Blinded at 63, I Can Still Learn," *Music Educators Journal* 58 (April 1972): 58-60.

Suite. The words she sang were "Gwen is walking well today," and so she was![4]

Music and art have been used together as a therapeutic technique in Vienna. Professor Berta Ernst uses music with painting or drawing in the treatment of handicapped or emotionally disturbed people.[5] In her sessions she asks for creative interpretation of musical works--single movements of absolute music or program music. Other activities include line drawing representing musical embellishments, or painting based on devices such as legato and staccato.

Movement and music involve perception and participation. Through movement, a person learns how and where to move the parts of the body that can be moved, thereby increasing body awareness, motor control, and coordination. Locomotive skills will be in accordance with present physical abilities, but music can be used to assist in two ways: (1) as an aid to movement, and (2) to create an atmosphere that can be expressed in movement.

Although music is no wonder drug, it can often be the means by which the patient may be calmed enough to be able to face the future. The choice of music for achieving this tranquillizing effect depends on each individual. Generally speaking, familiar music helps people to forget the present and remember happier days, although others reduce the tensions of a current situation by listening intently to a completely unknown work. Under ideal conditions, these people have a cassette tape recorder and headphones so that they may listen to their choice of music without disturbing others. The recorder and headphones should be placed where the person can operate it with a minimum of effort--day or night. A therapist could consult each person and ascertain if he would like to have a tape made. The patient should then have a period of time (a week is sufficient) to consider what he prefers to put on the tape. The tape should then be made as soon as the works are selected.

Contact with people who are suffering from dementia may be made through a program of Reality Orientation, which is a technique designed to be used with people exhibiting confused or

---

[4]"Case Study Using Music," *New Zealand Society for Music Therapy Newsletter* 3 (March 1980):3-4.

[5]"Report from Mary Edwards," *New Zealand Society for Music Therapy Newsletter* 3, no. 1 (March 1980):4-9.

disoriented behavior.[6] The purpose of reality orientation is to reverse or halt confusion, social withdrawal, and apathy characteristics of aging people.

The following is the basis of a schedule for a series of sixteen sessions of thirty minutes duration for a group of about eight people:

1. Daily therapy sessions should begin with oral communication of group members' names, then days of the week, months of the year, etc. In some cases, this will be followed by the individual's desire to write again and, in others, to read again

2. Pictures and poetry can be used as well as the reading of short stories about the topic being worked on in the session

3. The group members should be able to identify themselves and the therapist by name by the end of the first session

4. Everyone should be able to identify each other by name by the end of the third session

This emphasis on identifying people continues until, by the end of the eighth session, group members should be able to identify immediate members of the family by name and also be able to place them within the family, e.g., spouse, children, sister, etc. This identification process is more effective if the actual people are present, although it can be done by means of photographs.

The attention of the group members is now brought to bear on their surroundings so that, by the end of the fourteenth session, they should be able to identify the town (or city) they live in and describe certain aspects about it. If they live in an institution, they should know its name and where their room is in the complex. The aim, at the end of the sixteenth session, is that all group members should be able to demonstrate the ability to identify correctly all information covered during the program.

Music activities helpful to this program include listening to and discussing music written about a particular topic such as the weather, flowers, or the first name of a group member. Active music making is to be encouraged. The following three activities are enjoyable ways to support a program of this kind.

---

[6]Jennifer Riegler, "On Reality Orientation," *Journal of Music Therapy* 17 (Spring 1980):26-33.

Activity 1

Singing

This activity is especially effective if a group member recalls a tune from the past, or if the songs that are chosen contain a group member's name, e.g., "I Dream of Jeannie with the Light Brown Hair" or "Billy Boy." Other effective techniques include the singing of jingles about the day, date, weather, or simple T.V. jingles familiar to group members.

Humming, singing, even singing "la la" to well-known songs of their generation are splendid preliminary exercises for loosening the tongue and throat muscles and for bringing the voice forward in preparation for the oral communication of the lessons.

Activity 2

Playing Rhythm Instruments

Rhythmic accompaniment can support the songs and jingles. The rhythm instruments should be many and varied. They can be purchased or homemade. The reasons for using rhythm instruments are also many and varied. Some group members begin with a drum, triangle, or tambourine, using whole shoulder movements and, through perseverance and practice, are able to manage the fine finger control of castanet playing in a remarkably short time. Improvement that has been noted ranges from randomly striking a chime bar or drum to striking the instrument on the beat.

Other group members have been observed just banging the instruments on the table. In this situation, it is tempting to take the instruments from them; but before doing so, bear in mind that this uncontrolled activity may be one of the few ways these people can release feelings of frustration.

Activity 3

Turning Music "Outside-In"

Arrange for the group to move outside and experience the sounds around them. When they come back indoors, ask them to talk about their experience and, if they wish, to imitate the sounds they heard, either vocally or on a percussion instrument.

If the sessions are held indoors, arrange the group in a circle or semicircle rather than in rows. Whenever possible, however, take the group outside. The outdoors reactivates the senses of seeing, smelling, feeling, and especially hearing.

Begin the outdoor session on the veranda or in the garden. Then, with assistants to help with transportation, arrange to visit other places to gather new sounds. Places like the park, the pet shop, and the street provide interesting sounds.

Conclusion

How can we rehabilitate the handicapped? By educating society, by training therapists, and by encouraging the handicapped to try to reach their individual goals in life. The education of society is underway and therapists in many fields are being trained. The encouragement of the handicapped to try to fulfill their objectives must be the aim of empathetic friends and relatives with whom they come in contact. In all rehabilitation programs, music has proved to be a major ingredient of success.

REFERENCES

"Case Study Using Music." *New Zealand Society for Music Therapy Newsletter* 3 (March 1980):3-4.

Counsell, Alan. *So Clear in My Mind*. London: Hutchinson, 1982.

Dickie, Dale P. "Activities to Put Music in the Lives of the Elderly." New Zealand, 1982. (This paper may be obtained from the Education Advisor, New Zealand Council for Recreation and Sport, P.O. Box 5122, Wellington, New Zealand.)

Lipman, Miriam H. "Blinded at 63, I Can Still Learn." *Music Educators Journal* 58 (April 1972):58-60.

"Report from Mary Edwards." *New Zealand Society for Music Therapy Newsletter* 3, no. 1 (March 1980):4-9.

Riegler, Jennifer. "On Reality Orientation." *Journal of Music Therapy* 17 (Spring 1980):26-33.

A VERY SPECIAL ARTS PROGRAM: A MODEL FOR THE SYSTEMATIC DISSEMINATION OF INFORMATION ON ARTS WITH THE HANDICAPPED

by

EUGENE MAILLARD and JOANNE GRADY

The basis for the mission of Very Special Arts (formerly National Committee, Arts with the Handicapped) is to ensure that quality arts experiences are accessible to *all* persons, able and disabled. This policy was formulated during the 1974 National Conference on Arts and the Handicapped. The conference, funded by the Joseph P. Kennedy, Jr. Foundation, was coordinated by the Education Committee of the John F. Kennedy Center for the Performing Arts. Motivated by the needs of their various constituencies, and stimulated by this meeting, leaders in the fields of health, education, and the arts, as well as representatives of the federal government, sought to address the issue of arts accessibility; thus, the nucleus of the Very Special Arts was formed. With funding from the Kennedy Foundation and the U.S. Department of Health, Education, and Welfare, the Committee set out to unify the nation's efforts in this area. They planted the seeds of information from which a major national movement for arts with the handicapped has sprung.

The concept of the Very Special Arts (VSA) Program was developed by the original founders as an effective vehicle by which information and programming concerning arts and disabled persons could be systematically disseminated. The VSA Program is designed as an ongoing program, integrating the arts into the education of all disabled students. Its objective is to provide a noncompetitive opportunity for disabled students to celebrate and share their accomplishments in the visual and performing arts as a means of entering the mainstream of cultural and educational activity. Handicapped people of all ages who participate in VSA programs are offered a rich array of experiences to help them develop critical academic, social, and emotional skills. Arts education in the VSA manner is part of the general education of handicapped children and its aim is to develop the youngsters' personal artistic responsiveness and general learning. The program has grown from an initial festival in 1975 to more than 500 program sites in all fifty states, the District of Columbia, and Puerto Rico. In addition, there are program affiliates in forty nations.

By assisting with technical and management training, the VSA Program provides a unified identity for many local programs, thus strengthening their efforts. Important to the success of the program is the in-service training of VSA personnel. Very Special Arts staff and experts from the fields of education, arts, public information, and business meet annually with all VSA program coordinators to impart creative ways of expanding educational and instructional opportunities for handicapped people.

VSA program activities also involve parents, siblings, and the community at large. The highlight of a full year's arts programming comes with a culminating Very Special Arts Festival--a joyous celebration of the arts that includes workshops, demonstrations, exhibits, and performances given by students, arts educators, classroom teachers, and artists. The festivals are well attended, stimulate public interest in the arts with disabled persons, and create opportunities for all to admire the education and artistic accomplishments of others.

From the beginning, VSA felt that their priority was with fieldwork that had already begun and was being implemented, rather than turning attention to the generation and dissemination of new programming or techniques in arts training. In 1977, the Model Site Program was developed in the United States in an effort to support exemplary arts programs that successfully involved disabled people. Comprehensive programs providing arts experiences for handicapped persons served as demonstration and resource sites and provided replicable examples for programming throughout the U.S. Each Model Site was staffed by skilled professionals who provided technical assistance to other arts educators, special education instructors, parents, and other concerned individuals. The scope of each program was supported and documented in publications, films, and videotapes that were disseminated and replicated by the VSA program network. The results of these projects remain in the VSA resource library, available to all people in this field.

At the same time, the Special Projects Program was also developed as an information-gathering process. The program, conceived in response to the identified needs of VSA constituents, focused on the development of unique and innovative research projects, awareness projects, curriculum materials, teacher training, and other innovative arts-related projects. The Special Projects became effective national catalysts for program growth, innovation, and awareness since they function as resources for programs needing information and technical assistance.

The VSA-sponsored Model Sites and Special Projects in the United States were catalysts in establishing a national network of arts programming for disabled persons. In the later 1970s, in an effort to identify what work was already being done and to foster a greater national awareness, VSA tapped the existing energy and resources available, regardless of their relation to the VSA Program. With that accomplishment to their credit, VSA recently adopted a more streamlined approach to the gathering of information. Today, the results of current special-model projects are being fed directly into the VSA system as models for replication. VSA believes that our constituency will be better served if efforts are made national, and if these efforts are unified by integration into the main dissemination mechanism--the VSA Program.

From these beginnings, the VSA Program has continued to expand and to involve a wide range of disciplines, professions, agencies, and organizations across a vast area. The VSA Program acts as an effective networking device since it is the "common denominator" for all factions involved. This broad-reaching program requires and draws from the resources of many organizations and disciplines while at the same time serving as a link to the national and international organization. The VSA Program is a unique and proven method of providing arts opportunities for disabled populations. In a time of heightened awareness of the issues of the handicapped and cutbacks in funding, many museums, schools, government agencies, labor unions, and other organizations who have always been a resource for the nondisabled find it effective, efficient, and financially productive to affiliate with an established program like the VSA. By assisting us--i.e., through funding and program development--in our efforts to integrate disabled students into the mainstream of society, such groups have the benefit of addressing a broader, more far-reaching constituency.

The best instrument available for measuring the success of the VSA Program and other VSA arts programs is the resultant anecdotal data of "success stories" gathered over the past decade. The positive information available has proven that our concept has been effective in the classroom and has done much to increase the credibility of our program. By spreading the simple message that the arts "work," VSA can increase the priority given to arts with the handicapped in our networks of concern and, in turn, prioritize this issue in the minds of the American population at large.

Congress officially sanctioned the work of VSA as an important endeavor and thereby designated VSA as the nation's coordinating agency for the development and implementation of arts programs for all disabled individuals. Together with the passing by Congress of additional legislation concerning issues of accessibility and equal education for the handicapped, this endorsement has proven to be a powerful tool in broadening our scope of influence in schools, museums, and other public institutions across the country. In addition, there is great advantage to being an educational affiliate of the nation's cultural center, the John F. Kennedy Center for the Performing Arts. This association signifies to many that the mission of VSA is based on a culturally sound and timely concept. Powered by such support, VSA may confidently and successfully garner the participation and support of the public and private sectors. This has enabled VSA to take a leadership role in the field of arts education for the handicapped in our country.

Funding from the federal government as well as the private sector enables VSA to develop and implement arts programming. Because of its unique educational thrust, VSA, since its inception, has received the support of the United States government. In addition, VSA is an international program that draws support from the private sector. Private corporations have found that they can experience meaningful involvement and be cast in a favorable light when they are involved in flourishing VSA programs. VSA has been successful in uniting these two avenues of support. This has been a crucial factor in the growth and maintenance of the funding base and a key to the program's success, since one sector fosters the support of the other and assists in perpetuating an even greater public awareness.

The favorable participation of the media has also been vital to the past successes of VSA. Very Special Arts was most fortunate through the years in enlisting the cooperation of the mass media. Several different tactics have been used to accomplish this. VSA has been able to attract public attention not only by sponsoring innovative programs but also by working to promote them with the assistance of nationally recognized spokespersons. Many celebrities, professional artists, and government leaders have participated in special national events, in local Very Special Arts Festivals, and by endorsing VSA via public service announcements for national or local print and broadcast. These components are combined in the VSA National Awareness Program. The Program is designed to stimulate public interest in the activities of VSA and to promote the concept of utilizing the arts to enhance the lives of disabled people throughout the world. Since the VSA network now encompasses all fifty states and affiliates in forty nations, informed and concerned citizens can easily become involved in local VSA activities in their area. Positive and widespread media coverage of the local and international activities of VSA has been very important in securing the support of the private sector for whom favorable public exposure is important.

One of the goals of VSA is to expand international awareness and to provide a system for sharing information about existing programs in the arts for disabled persons. As a result of the impact that this programming and information network has made in the United States, the Committee has made an effort to exchange information with other countries and to share adaptive arts activities that enhance learning and enrich the lives of handicapped individuals.

Very Special Arts has taken a broad approach in attempting to form an international network of arts with the handicapped organizations. Since 1982, VSA has participated in several conferences on arts and the handicapped in Latin America. In June 1983, VSA co-hosted an international conference in Vienna, Austria that was attended by leaders throughout Europe in the field of arts and education with the handicapped. Once again, there was an attempt to investigate the needs of the disabled and of work being done in the field--this time, on an international basis. Although no definite format for an international program was decided at the time, participants of the Vienna conference agreed that a vehicle for information exchange is essential for the future development of the field--not only for the countries that already have arts programs for the disabled but also to encourage those countries that have not yet begun programs to do so.

VSA hosted an International Seminar in Washington, D.C., May 1984, during the National Very Special Arts Festival. The Seminar also was in celebration of the tenth anniversary of Very Special Arts. More than one hundred and seventy delegates representing sixty-two nations met during the Seminar to share ideas and techniques regarding programs for disabled persons and to discuss the organization of an international exchange network in the field. Although it is evident that program implementation and administrative procedures vary from country to country, there is a marked similarity among the goals of arts for the handicapped programs and a common belief in the value of these programs for the social integration of disabled populations. Very Special Arts initiated an International Committee, Arts with the Handicapped, now called Very Special Arts International, in order to address common needs expressed by international participants at the Seminar. VSA International facilitates the international exchange of information and the expansion and promotion of arts programs with the handicapped all over the world. In response to the needs expressed by many international representatives during the Seminar, VSA International is initiating a series of international activities that foster a meaningful exchange of resources and information. VSA International feels that the information dissemination mechanism inherent in the VSA Program in the United States provides a model for nations interested in developing a similar Very Special Arts Program. VSA International works in cooperation with existing organizations and agencies to create a united international movement that will benefit not only these organizations but disabled populations throughout the world.

There are currently forty nations affiliated with this network. By so doing, national organizations have a greater opportunity to foster their nation's awareness of the benefits the arts provide towards integrating disabled individuals into the mainstream of society. Technical information on the implementation and promotion of arts programs with disabled populations and resources is being exchanged within the international network. National organizations benefit from inter-agency/international adaptive arts curricula. Furthermore, through this international network, guidance in the development of national plans and services for disabled populations can be given by other countries that have produced successful programs.

In the United States, similar local organizations gain prestige, credibility, and influence by affiliating with the national VSA Program. This same beneficial effect is possible at the international level. Small national efforts will be able to achieve more public awareness, benefit from the program developments in other nations, and stabilize their ability to attract federal support by identifying themselves as affiliates of Very Special Arts International, a worldwide union of professionals dedicated to working in this field.

As Mrs. Jean Kennedy Smith, VSA founder and Chairperson of the VSA Program, expressed in her address to the delegates at the International Seminar in Washington, D.C.: "We may be from different continents, different systems, different peoples, but we share a common quest . . . toward achieving the ideal that disabled people everywhere have the opportunity to learn and grow through the arts."

Today, there have been tremendous successes throughout the world. Twenty nations have had Very Special Arts Festivals of their own. Training has been conducted in many of the forty VSA International affiliate organizations. VSA International is working in collaboration with both public and private sector international agencies and corporations. There is a genuine global spirit committed to equality in the arts for all.

MUSIC AND WELL-BEING: VIEWING PHILOSOPHIES, TRAINING MODELS, AND OPERATIONAL PROCEDURES

by

RONALD D. PRICE, EILEEN F. REXROAD,
and KAY L. STEPHENS

Well-being requires that basic needs be satisfied. In addition to the general concern for physical well-being, equal attention must be given to the emotional, intellectual, social, aesthetic, and spiritual aspects of life. Since the human is a synergism, any condition that threatens the health of any component can indeed affect other areas as well.

Music has been a significant part of all cultures that have been studied. It may be concluded that there is a universal need for people to express themselves aesthetically. Such expression may transcend the limits of usual communication (speech, writing, gestures). Music embodies all that is unique to the human experience. Whether primitive (as noted by limitations in melodic, harmonic, structural, or textural components), or sophisticated (symphonic literature, chamber music, opera, jazz), the production or reception of music involves the transmission or communication of human thought and feeling through the auditory medium. The absence of an element, either sound or emotion, may negate the existence of music.

For those whose lives are affected by disabilities (whether endogenous or exogenous), chronic or terminal illness, the aging process, or environmental factors, the need for aesthetic expression exists. Because of the inherent qualities of music, it is both possible and desirable to develop opportunities by which participants can reconfirm their individuality and membership in the human community. Such experiences can, while focusing on aesthetic expression, serve to stimulate intellectual activity, social interaction, emotional stability, and spirituality. Fundamental to such a philosophy is the focus on healthy persons rather than healthy organisms.

Professional service musicians do and will continue to play a signficant role in the process of well-being. Music education and music therapy were once distinctly different in their purpose, procedures, and outcomes. However, increased awareness of professional service musicians enables one to conclude that, in any situation involving people and music, learning can occur, aesthetic response may be elicited, and extra-musical changes may be realized.

everything has a name and everything knows its place, and we can leverage very little. But in the time of parenthesis we have extraordinary leverage and influence--individually, professionally and institutionally--if we can only get a clear sense, a clear con- ception, a clear vision, of the road ahead.

My God, what a fantastic time to be alive![3]

---

[3]Naisbitt, p. 252.

REFERENCES

Kohut, Daniel L. *Musical Performance: Learning, Theory, and Pedagogy.* Englewood Cliffs, New Jersey: Prentice-Hall, 1984.

Naisbitt, John. *Megatrends.* New York: Warner Books, 1982.

MUSICAL PERSONALITY, THERAPY, AND WELL-BEING

by

PAMELA H. STEELE

In music therapy, the patient reveals his musical personality to the therapist in interactive music making. This paper will address the concept of "musical personality" and why it is believed that in encountering a musical personality, one encounters an essential aspect of a person. Also to be considered is how the therapist's discovery of a musical personality forms part of the process of therapy in which the patient moves towards his own rehabilitation and well-being. These ideas will be illustrated with case material of music therapy with a group of emotionally disturbed children, and one group member in particular.

The term "musical personality" refers to a person's disposition to behave musically in particular ways in response to musical experiences that involve listening, performing, composing, or improvising. This may be expressed as a preference for one piece of music, or type of music, over another. As performing musicians, we may find that in the interpretation of a piece some parts are quite unproblematic whereas others are less comfortable and have to be worked at, thought about, mused over, left, reconsidered, etc. This is not simply an issue of pure technical ability. As improvising musicians, we find that certain tempi, meters, rhythmic patterns, pitches, tones, and timbres are more natural and familiar to us than others, and that they recur in our playing. There may be an almost physical sense of discomfort when we push ourselves (or are pushed) into other tempi, just as when we have to walk faster than usual to keep up with an energetic friend.

Why do we think that musical personality is an essential part of a person? First, because music is a world-wide phenomenon whose primary elements (rhythm and pitch) are inherent in the human body. The body is periodic, functioning in daily, monthly, and longer cycles. Heartbeat is a basic pulse running through and fundamental to our lives even before birth. Our voices make pitched sounds when they cry, scream, laugh, gurgle, babble, and speak.

Furthermore, shared music making reveals *patterns of interaction* among those engaged in it. When the elements of such musical interaction, rhythm, and pitch are seen in the interactional context, *timing* between the players is observable and significant. Simultaneity, turn-taking, interruption, canon, etc., can be heard, as can imitation, variation, and repetition between

27

players. These features of interaction that are highlighted in music are features of human interaction from early mother-infant relationship, through preverbal babble, to use of verbal language itself. It may be that it is in the earliest stages that patterns of interaction are established that affect the later stages, and that it is in this early stage that music therapists must look for the foundation of musical personality.

The second reason musical personality is considered an essential part of a person is that it is not merely an expression of the musical knowledge or skill that a person has acquired. Rather, to be involved with music is to be involved in a process requiring what we may term "imagination," "creativity," or "the ability to play" (in the broadest sense of that word), whether we are listening to, or making music. There is a sensation of "ranging inwardly" that has an outer expression in active music making. The extent to which we are musicians, dancers, or painters depends not only on our technical abilities in each field but on the extent to which we can allow ourselves to explore and express our imaginative faculty for play.

This is sometimes referred to as the feeling content of music. Music arouses feelings in us, and we express feelings through music. This may be thought of in terms of a relatively simple emotion such as "anger," "sadness," "hopelessness," or, like the energetic friend who walks too fast for our comfort, music may give us a physical sensation, i.e., the hairs on our necks may rise, our hearts may pound. Music may evoke a visual image, thought, or memory--"feelings," therefore, in the broadest sense of that word.

Music therapy reveals the musical personality of the patient, his natural rhythms and pitches, his patterns of interaction, and his feelings. In group music therapy, the therapist repeatedly encounters the musical personalities of several patients as they reveal themselves in musical interaction, both with the therapist and with each other. In these musical relationships, as in any relationship, the consistency in each musical personality does not mean that the personality is incapable of change or that the same musical behavior can be expected every time. To deny this would be to fail to acknowledge the complexity and subtlety of all human interaction.

Peter, age seven, is a case in point. The limitations of this paper do not permit the full exploration of his musical relationships with other group members, although it should be remembered that to consider him as an isolated case is to abstract him somewhat artificially from the group setting. A brief account of the entire group will minimize this effect.

Casework

The group consisted of five emotionally disturbed children, ages six to nine. It was formed in January 1984 at St. Thomas' Psychiatric Day Hospital for children, and the members attended one morning or a whole day per week in order to work with two staff nurses trained in psychiatry. Their activities included painting, clay, stories, board games, and house play. Music therapy took place with the whole group (including staff) for a forty-minute session once a week. The group sat on the floor in a circle in a corner of a large and pleasant therapy room.

Musical activities of the group may be considered in four categories: drum improvisation, precomposed instrumental arrangements of songs, unaccompanied songs, and melodic improvisation.

Drum Improvisation

This occurred usually at the beginning of each session and was undirected in the sense that each person chose a drum and a beater, and the only instruction and direction from the therapist was "to play." However, in the ensuing improvisation, the therapist did sometimes present a musical idea that the group might adopt.

Out of this initial group improvisation, the therapist would suggest that one person play to another. Thus, "dialogue" grew between two players while the rest of the group listened or provided a rhythmic ostinato over which the dialogue could be heard.

These simple forms and variations of them consistently provided a medium for the rhythmic life of the group. This activity also allowed the therapist to become acquainted with each individual and with the cohesiveness, or lack of it, of the group. These improvisations often began with an almost overwhelming feeling of chaos and mismatch, with children playing at different tempi from each other, some frequently changing tempi, changing meter, often playing very loudly, while others did not play at all or only sporadically.

Precomposed Instrumental Arrangements of Songs

The therapist presented song material arranged for various instrumental parts. Parts were allocated according to the abilities and desires of the children as the therapist perceived them to be, and, although the tempo, key, and individual parts were predetermined, impromptu variations were incorporated where appropriate.

Unaccompanied Songs

These were initially introduced as a "musical offering" from the therapist rather than with the intention of getting the children to sing. Without an instrumental accompaniment to distract them, the therapist's singing voice reached out to offer an experience of clarity and simplicity that required no activity on their part. As the sessions progressed, children did spontaneously join in with these songs.

Melodic Improvisation

The children played a xylophone, metallophone, or chime bars. This was a problematic area of music making until the nineteenth session. The chaotic character of the drum improvisation reappeared, with the added complication of different pitches being available to each child. Even when all the instruments were tuned to a scale in which all possible intervals are consonant, such as the pentatonic CDFGA, the strongly rhythmic use of melodic instruments without a shared pulse (and the addition of less strongly melodic instruments such as the triangle, frequently used in a markedly rhythmic way) led to an unsettling musical piece.

Significantly, it was through the drum improvisations that the group shared a basic pulse for the first time (in the nineteenth session). After this development, a theme played in melodic improvisation by the therapist allowed the other players to accompany, imitate, and vary it in their own playing, within a shared, basic beat.

Having thus evoked something of the group's musical personality and the forms through which it was expressed, let us now consider one member in more detail.

Peter was the younger of two brothers, aged nine and seven, both of whom attended the music therapy group. They lived with their mother, their father having been in prison since Peter was only a few months old. Larry, the elder, was initially referred because of enuresis and encopresis, cold sores on his face and body, and a general appearance of neglect, which resulted in his being bullied at school. He said he was very unhappy, felt unloved, and felt that everyone was against him. The community physician

30

described him as "severely depressed." When his treatment began, it became apparent that Peter too was eneuretic and appeared ill cared for and unhappy. He was described as being aggressive in school and as constantly arguing with his brother and mother at home. Peter was small for his age and often dressed in grubby, ill-fitting clothes. He had unkempt, dirty blond hair and an attractive but often pinched looking face.

From the first session, his drum playing was characterized by fast beats; a loud dynamic; a regular meter; and an absence of rests and, therefore, no rhythmic pattern. These features created a perseverative, isolated quality in his playing.

He would choose the biggest drum and a hard wooden stick, sometimes moving his whole body to achieve maximum physical force. There was drive and energy in the playing, which was matched by two other boys'; but because their playing had different rhythmic features, the effect was chaotic. At times Peter seemed completely self-absorbed, then would appear to direct his torrent of playing towards the group, sometimes laughing and appearing almost defiant.

This tendency to direct outwards became marked in session seven, when he chose to play in dialogue to Larry. As the dialogue progressed, Peter playing much as described, his parts became longer and longer so that all sense of dialogue was eventually lost. He had become a soloist, forcing an audience (Larry) to listen. He played with the wrong end of the stick; played the underside of the drum; wrote on the drum with the stick as if it were a pen; karate-chopped the drum with his left hand while beating with the stick in his right; tapped and rattled the sides of the drum; and scratched the skin with his fingernails. All this was done in an energetic, almost frantic way, while he gazed intently into Larry's face. At moments, he would make a ritardando and diminuendo as if he were going to stop. Then, as Larry prepared to play, he would resume his flood of beating, as before. In the following sessions, he almost always chose to play to Larry and did so in a similar way.

He carried the prevailing character of his drum work over onto melodic instruments. Rather than explore their melodic qualities, he played the metallophone so hard that its tone was deadened by the hammer effect of his stick, producing metallic bangs with only a trace of pitch and tone in them. He played in a continuous, fast, basic beat using notes of equal length with no rests at fixed tempo.

Vocally, he either made unvoiced sounds (clicks, raspberries, etc.) or sang in a monotone. On days when he seemed particularly distressed, he would begin singing with the group, then sing continuously, with no rests between phrases, lines, or verses, so that he arrived at the end when everyone else was still in the middle. Sometimes he would disguise his voice with a sneering, mocking tone. It was clear, however, from the beginning, that he was held by melody and by the therapist's singing voice, even if only in a brief moment of stillness and listening.

In summary, Peter's musical personality in active music making revealed itself in loud, fast playing; without rests or variation; and in unclearly pitched, unresonant sounds. However, when he managed simply to listen to singing, he could appreciate other tempi and dynamics, truly melodic phrases, and clear pitches, even if he was not actively engaged in performing. In the precomposed instrumental arrangement of songs, he experienced obvious frustration or anxiety while playing simple parts that required other tempi or the observation of rests. He therefore gave the impression of lacking simple skills of memory or motor control. This musical personality had the effect, therefore, of isolating him from any group musical experiences that required anything other than the musical behavior already described.

Rehabilitation and Well-Being

How is it, then, that the expression of musical personality is part of the process of therapy? In music therapy, the capacity of music to express feeling and to reveal primary patterns of interaction is employed by the patient in the therapeutic environment whose limits are safeguarded by the therapist. The patient and therapist jointly create music in musical interaction. The therapist takes as the starting point the musical personality of the patient and, in this case, that of the group.

There is acknowledgement of the significance and validity of the child's musical personality and the abilities and feelings it expresses through what may be described as music therapy techniques. These may be considered under four headings: (1) listening; (2) reflecting back; (3) creating a musical context, a significant part of which is the patient's music; and (4) bringing variety.

The first technique involves listening to the others' music. This is attentive listening that allows the therapist to hear its qualities of tempo, pitch, tone, timbre, etc.

The second technique involves reflecting back on those qualities in one's own music making.

In the third technique, there is a musical context created, of which the patient's music is a significant part. The music shared by the patient and therapist has not only the qualities of the patient's music but also the qualities of the therapist's musical personality as it expresses itself in response to that patient.

The fourth technique is one of bringing variety into the qualities of the shared music, by virtue of the therapist being a music maker who acknowledges and affirms the musical personality of another, but is not taken over by it.

In group music therapy, each patient should have the experience of being musically acknowledged without feeling that his music alone dominates the group music. This experience is afforded by the therapist and by each member, one to another. So, too, the musical personality of the group should be acknowledged without the therapist failing to introduce musical qualities that it does not yet have or has not yet revealed.

Through these primary experiences of being affirmed, held, and withstood that are afforded by the medium of music in the therapeutic environment, the patient can move towards his own rehabilitation and a state of greater well-being. The therapist does not rehabilitate the patient by observing the manifestations of his musical personality and setting about to change them. Rather, the patient's musical personality, once affirmed and withstood, can change and grow within the musical relationship(s).

Within the music therapy environment, Peter's well-being was seen to be limited in his relationship with his brother; his relationship with other group members; and in what we may call "the quality of his inner life," or "feeling life," as this was revealed through his driven and unrelenting playing. His playing had different qualities, however, by the nineteenth session when, during the group drum improvisation, Peter shared a steady rhythmic motif in a slower tempo than usual for him, sustaining attention and involvement through the playing and the rests. Later, in a male-female dialogue, Peter, his brother, and another boy shared strong, unified playing of a rhythmic motif that Peter sustained while the other two occasionally subdivided the basic beats in a potentially unsettling way. All this playing was improvised.

His drum dialogues with Larry have continued much as described. Their relationship, however, has developed through singing. During the fifteenth session, when we worked on a West

Indian call and response song, "Hill 'n Gully Rida," Peter asked if he and Larry could sing the call to the rest of the group, and then did so. By the twentieth session, they reached a high point of co-activity in this kind of activity when they sustained their part together and negotiated an accelerando and ritardando that the group had to follow, a musical feat requiring considerable mutuality, sensitivity, and skill.

Peter's voice has become fuller in tone and, at times, more clearly pitched. During the fourteenth session, as the therapist improvised vocally in a song ("Sammy Dead") that was familiar to them, Peter began to join in, improvising clearly pitched melodic lines in a committed and intense way, his eyes shut and his face tipped upwards. At other times, he would stretch out on the floor, either just listening or sometimes singing in a soft and tuneful voice and staring into space.

Rehabilitation is a process not of invention but of restoration. We need not say that Peter's musical personality has changed from having one set of characteristics to another. Perhaps he is engaged in a process of rediscovering aspects of himself that have been occluded by the prevalence of his loud, perseverative, isolated musical personality, a process that has been facilitated by the opportunity to express that limited musical personality and have it acknowledged in a therapeutic environment.

In conclusion, two questions may be raised that are suggested by work with this group: (1) What place, if any, has verbal language in music therapy? and (2) What part does the therapist's musical personality play in the therapeutic process?

In answer to the first question, the three foundation stones on which Peter's music therapy stands are: (1) his past, where patterns of interaction were established; (2) his everyday life, where the expression of his personality results in problematic behavior within family and school relationships; and (3) his experience of himself and others in the therapeutic environment. Is it necessary that he consciously make links between these three aspects of his life in order for him to receive daily benefit?

Must he be able to address himself to the origins of his limitations by relating them to his past, and must he be able in turn to relate this to his everyday life? Indeed, must he even be aware, at a conscious level, that he has problems? One of the strengths of music therapy is that in revealing oneself musically, the patient communicates in a way that may be considered an unconscious rather than conscious level. Does this very point, however, limit the scope of music therapy to facilitate a patient's move towards well-being?

The question of the place of language in music therapy can be answered only by taking the lead from the patient and the needs he demonstrates. Some changes in musical personality have already been described. Peter has rarely introduced verbal language, but when he has, its use has been striking. Once, when beating the drum in his characteristic way and holding it up in the air, he began to beat it with his head. When he stopped, he told us that he bangs his head against the wall at home and at school. When the therapist remarked that this must be very painful, he said: "No, it's not; I don't feel it at all." His drum playing was like the head banging: perseverative, angry, violent, but now not only self-directed. Certainly, his musical personality had a deadened, anesthetized quality.

During the twenty-fourth session, we sang a song about an evil spirit, Jumbie, whom people blame when things go wrong. When the therapist asked the group to suggest additional verses, Peter became very excited and said: "Jumbie steals all the bed, steals all the light, pours water on the fuses and the lights go off." He then insisted that we incorporate these ideas in the verses. The hospital personnel know that Peter's mother, who supports her boys on welfare, encourages them to sleep in her bed, and she often switches off lights, heating, and the stove in order to save electricity. Peter obviously wanted to make connections between his everyday life and the therapeutic environment. It is questionable whether the music therapist has either the opportunity or skill at such times to help him to explore fully his incipient insights.

The second question suggested by this group therapy asks what part the therapist's musical personality plays in the therapeutic process. It is not possible any more than it is desirable that musical interaction take place without the expression of the therapist's own musical personality. It is necessary, however, that the situation is not used to fulfill the therapist's own musical needs and that she can contain her musical response to the patient's musical personality.

Many music therapists are themselves patients in psychotherapy, and all are musicians who will to some extent have been made aware of their musical personality in the course of their musical experience. However, it may be that music therapists should themselves be patients in music therapy in order to most appropriately and usefully acquaint themselves with their musical personality.

One striking feature of the work with this group has been the strong emotional change running through the music we have shared. At certain moments, the therapist felt the emotional impact so strongly that it required conscious effort, sometimes retrospectively, to establish the musical phenomena that transmitted it. As music therapists, we are often called upon to give accounts of our work and frequently find ourselves using the terminology of fields such as physiology, psychology, or education to describe what, after all, we as musicians experience and respond to as primarily musical phenomena. If I have underemphasized the feeling content of interactional music therapy, it has been in an attempt to return to the primary data of the therapeutic relationship--those of the musical phenomena, the expressions of musical personality.

MUSIC AND THE BODY

by

JACQUELINE VERDEAU-PAILLÈS

Music and body movement constitute a form of expression through rhythm, motion, and melody. The classical clinical approach never provided us with the kind of insight into our patients' personalities that is now available through music and expressive bodily movement. Through music and body movement we have a broad basis for analysis, an easier mode of communication, and a method for encouraging creativity and mobilizing energy.

Expression therapy, grounded in listening, improvisation, and body movement, is not limited to the psychiatrist's domain. This therapeutic mode is also important for the therapist whose patients are suffering from disorders involving anxiety, blocking, and fatalistic notions. The approach, of course, is not new, but rather in a constant state of being rediscovered. We are attempting to free the technique from past practices, keeping one foot in our own heritage and the other in new cultures and methods that are regularly examined and submitted to critical analysis. It is our task to subsume the new information into our existing body of knowledge and understanding. The patient and therapist are now partners in a contract based on a new kind of relationship and exchange.[1]

Most therapeutic techniques using music and body movement take the patient back to a point in the past, a situation in which sound, body, and movement are linked. There cannot be any duality between the body and the mind. We must at all times grasp the individual in his totality, involving the body in our understanding of the patient, remembering that his listening, his expressiveness, and his creativity work through the body.

The Link Between Sound and Movement

The link between sound and movement is a close one and can be proven scientifically. The study of anatomy shows us the only example of an organ that is at once sensorial and motoric: the

---

[1]Jacqueline Verdeau-Paillès, *La musique et l'expression corporelle en thérapeutique psychiatrique* (Paris: Masson, 1982), p. 12.

eighth cranial pair that serves both as the auditory nerve and the balance nerve.

Comparative embryology shows the human brain as the result of a combination of different brains. The most primitive one is the reptilian brain, a source of elementary behaviors. Next we have the limbic brain (one we hold in common with the lower mammalian species) superimposed on the reptilian brain. The limbic brain is activated by the simultaneous appearance of sound perception and movement, and it can be considered as the base of affective and motoric activity.

The third brain, which covers the other two, is a characteristic of the human species. It is the cerebral crust, and it matures much later. It is this brain that permits the acquisition of language, specialized movement, and the development of musical sense. Any breakdowns during this evolutionary process may induce disorders.

The study of human development lends further proof to the existence of a tight link between sound and motor activity. Scientific studies of fetal movement during the intra-uterine stage and then of the reactions of this same being as a newborn tend to demonstrate the influence of sudden movements and violent sounds to which the mother was submitted during pregnancy.

Newborn children have been calmed by: (1) the mother's heartbeat recorded through a liquid environment--the same condition in which the fetus originally heard the sound; (2) the rhythm of a lullaby that recalls the pendular motion of the pregnant mother's heavy gait; (3) a particular musical work or works of the same composer that were listened to frequently by the pregnant mother.

Similar experiences such as those cited above have given credence to hypotheses that, in turn, have developed into therapuetic positions in the area of obstetrical gynecology as well as the field of pediatric and adult psychology. For example, Bertrand has used this approach in parturition techniques, while Benenzon has attempted the opening of communication channels with autistic children through sound and movement.

A new branch of neurophysiology examines musical behavior in relation to the cerebral structures. Neurologists in the past could localize the motor centers by studying their lesions. Thanks to the study of aphasia, language centers in the brain were pinpointed. The clinical electroencephalographic and radiological examinations of patients suffering from amusia have also enabled us to determine the cerebral seat of musical functions and the connections between these centers.

Because of its universality, ethnomusicology is helpful in learning more about the developmental process. In earliest history, the cries, moans, and calls of primitive man preceded language. In the beginning, it was an unconnected sequence of sounds that expressed pleasure, pain, and danger. Melody came from the imitation of bird songs, the babbling of brooks, the breaking of waves, and the rustling of leaves. Rhythm, however, preceded all of these things. Ethnomusicology presents music as the mirror of corporal movement. In the words of J. Blacking, "Very often, the expressive aim of the musical work must be investigated through an identification with the corporal movements that originated it, and the origin of these movements can be found in culture as well as in the individual's particularities."[2]

Sound and Music, Gesture and Body Expressions
Common Components

Rhythm

Rhythm activates the musical phenomenon. It confers upon music its temporal unity (through which music exists); it is the actual life of music, that aspect of music that continually flows on. Rhythm is also the realization of shapes generated by movement. Like a flowing river, rhythm is also a wave, a shape in time. The association of both concepts imparts to musical rhythm the sense of an irreversible unfolding at which time identifiable and signifying movements take shape. Time in which rhythm flourishes is a reality that is very near that psychic space in which levels of sound take on a certain meaning. As a movement in psychical space cannot occur without generating a psychical time, one can likewise reason that sonorous shape and musical time constitute a unique psychic whole, spatial and temporal at the same time.[3]

Rhythm is the sequence and the proportion of durations. It is, in the broadest sense, musical movement as a whole. Music does not exist in immobility. Rhythm is the temporal condition of acts

---

[2]J. Blacking, *How Musical Is Man?* (London: Faber & Faber, 1976), p. 112.

[3]D. Porte, *Science de la musique* (Paris: Bordas, 1977), pp. 902-6.

that are executed in and unable to exist without sonorous space. Its actual existence presupposes movement, and its organization presupposes periodicity, at least in the first rhythmic shapes. It has been said that Vincent D'Indy summarized the essence of rhythm by describing it as order and proportion in space and time.[4] This definition allows us to conceive the interdependence between the organic rhythms and those that are outside the individual.

Rhythm also exists in body movements and their sequence. The genetic conception of rhythm places the rhythmic cell in a prominent position as the first unit, an energic temporal whole of two opposite forces.[5] Our perception of psychical time is generated by our consciousness of the vital cadences inside ourselves. The basic modules of rhythm are heart throbs, respiratory movements, and the rhythms of walk and gestures. It is by means of cadence--the first of all rhythmical realities--that man expresses the consciousness of his own existence. This consciousness is expressed in corporal space by dance and in sonorous space by music.

The first examples of basic rhythms are found in the corporal area. The binary cadence, for example, is the cadence of gait; the ternary cadence, one of respiration. In this second cadence, expiration is twice as long as inspiration, the time factor made possible only through the interrelationship of the two. Complex rhythmic organization is simply different combinations of binary and ternary rhythms. The conductor Ernest Ansermet developed the cadential conception of rhythm, a notion that is at once opposed and complementary to the metric conception. The metric conception, a more formal approach, contributes nothing to our understanding and fails to explain the part rhythm plays in the affective power of music. If the movement of sounds in time affects us, it is because this movement is, above all, the external manifestation of an interior energy that is in itself cadential.[6]

The fact that an organism presents an ensemble of rhythmical functions, that musical rhythm and its organization affect us because they are in tune with our own internal rhythm, must not make us rush to the conclusion that the origin of musical rhythm

---

[4]Ibid., p. 905.

[5]Ibid.

[6]E. Ansermet, *Les fondements de la musique dans la conscience humaine*, 2 vols. (Neuchatel: La Baconnière, 1961), 1:205.

can be found in organic rhythms. There are interesting relationships between the two, but a direct correlation must not be inferred. It is possible to suspect a correlation between the respiratory rhythm of a man at rest and the coming and going of waves. In fact, poems and lullabies often speak of this analogy. It has been noticed, despite the performance practices of many conductors, that Beethoven indicated 80 (a normal heart rhythm) as the metronomic tempo of the "Hymn to Joy" in the Ninth Symphony. This observation should not lead us to a specious inference. What is far more certain is that tempo corresponds to the internal sense of the existential cadence and of the organization of cadences. The existential cadential unit could be represented either by heart rhythm or by the rhythm of a fast or slow gait.

Harmonic music and our own internal rhythms achieve a kind of synergism in the following situations: (1) an andante is the melodic cadence, that which palpitates within us--our inner life; (2) the allegro is sustained by this existential melodic cadence--it is the superstructure; and (3) the adagio in turn presents the melodic cadence as a superstructure of the existential cadence.

Furthermore, these tempo indications are given in terms of movement: andante, a moderate pace; allegro, a rapid and gay movement; adagio, a slow and comfortable movement or the slowing down of the basic tempo in the execution of the work. These few reflections on tempo have their application in therapy.

Melody and Harmony

Melody is defined as a succession of musical sounds of different levels. It is the horizontal aspect of a classical musical text. Harmony is characterized by the formation and concatenation of an ensemble of simultaneous sounds. This simultaneity is the vertical aspect of the musical text. Although melody finds its beginnings in the amplification of speech, it is dance that very quickly supplies both with rhythmic support. Moreover, just as there is often a rhythm that sustains a melody, so one can also find a melody in rhythmic compositions. Rhythm generates movement.

And do we not at the same time hear of balance in motoric activity and lack of balance within movement?

Vibration

J. J. Matras defines musical sound as a very rapid sinusoidal vibrating movement limited by superior audibility thresholds to a frequency of about 20,000 periods per second. Frequencies lower than fifteen vibrations per second are no longer perceived as sound levels; when they are lower than ten, they become rhythmic pulsations.[7]

Vibration is a network of rapid periodic movements. Rhythm and melody have a common nature: they are vibratory movements of variable frequency considered by acousticians as the transmission of a mechanical energy. There may be an infinite number of vibratory associations since the body perceives them with different perception thresholds, which depend in turn on individual receptivity, posture, and the position of the body in relation to the source of the sound.

The physical side of music depends on the variable resonance of the different parts of the body in response to the amplitude and frequency of the vibratory stimulus, the direction taken by the sound inside the body, the state of tension or relaxation of the listener, and on the duration of the vibratory effect.

Somatic effects of vibrations can also be measured. In doing so, we extend the meaning of the physical phenomenon of resonance to the area of receptivity to music. Resonance is the scientific aspect of what the musician calls "sympathetic vibration." In more precise terms, it is that ability of the body to vibrate spontaneously when vibratory waves of identical, multiple, or sub-frequencies are broadcast near it. We can now make the analogy that we resonate with music when melody, rhythm, tempo, and affective quality correspond with our inner being. It is at this point that therapy is achieved.

Vibrations have their greatest impact when musicians use a technique known as vibrato. Vibrato gives a richer expressiveness to sound through a mixing of harmonics with tightly linked sounds. The violinist obtains vibrato through a movement of the fifth finger and a rapid back-and-forth motion of the wrist. The cellist, on the other hand, uses a movement of the forearm to get the same effect. Vibrato is also possible with wind instruments if special breathing techniques are used. The singer uses the vibrato technique in order to gain a greater sonority. To achieve this state, the singer must be completely supple so that the body can vibrate

---

[7]J. J. Matras, *Le son* (Paris: Que sais-je? - P.U.F., 1967), p. 82.

totally. The well-disciplined vibrato is obtained through a light and rapid movement of the sound at the top, making the voice more fascinating and expressive.

Sound can bring about a sensation of fullness both to the performer and listener. This is a state that overcomes a person almost imperceptibly, developing only when he interacts with the music. The individual identifies with and turns into it, existing both in the past and the present, and perceiving only his inner reaction. Gregorian Chant, for example, seems to come from everywhere and nowhere at the same time; reverberating on the walls, the floor, and the vaults of a cathedral; encircling the listener; and filling him completely. It is then that music is experienced physically as a body tension, and the internal feelings generated can be expressed in movements.

Tension/Relaxation: Opposites

If opposition is the essential element of all musical meaning, it is also the groundwork of our body rhythms and movements. Jacques Chailley expounded on Stavinsky's axiom by showing that the major value of a musical work and its impact comes from the delicate balance between yielding to the anticipated relaxation and tensing up for the next part.[8] The concept of dynamic equilibrium is the result of the opposition between the opposing forces of tension and relaxation. This notion of opposing forces is true in Western, Eastern, and Far-Eastern musical systems. The music of ancient China is based on the principles of peace/quiet and energy/aggression.

Vital functions of the body are cadences based on this same principle: the systolic/diastolic beating of the heart, the inspiration/expiration of respiration, the lifting and setting down of the feet during walking, and the tension/relaxation of our movements. Although contemporary artistic and therapeutic techniques must hold on to those elements of classical dance that impart elegance, rhythm, and harmony of movement, we must nevertheless recognize the doors that have been opened in modern dance by Isadora Duncan, Ted Shawn, Martha Graham, and many others. Through expressive and creative dances, these individuals develop movements wherein the body expresses life itself, with an expression devoid of artifice and stamped with a rare intensity. The entire body participates, exploits the physiological rhythms, and

---

[8]J. Chailley, "Essai sur les structures mélodiques," *Revue de Musicologie* 44 (1959):139-75.

incessantly develops the opposing forces of tension and relaxation. The dancer accepts the weight of her body, no longer refusing the relationship to the ground upon which she treads barefoot. No longer is she an unreal being, part of a romantic dream, a Pavlova seeming to float as she dances Giselle. Rather, she is a human being like those who are participating in the experience either by watching her or joining in the dance. The dancer has now become one with the music and its elements. We have taken the arts to a point that will serve as the basis of our therapeutic efforts.

Silence is an extension of this concept of opposites. The silence that follows music is different from the expectant silence that preceded it. This consequent silence supports movement, facilitates listening, and prepares us to communicate. Claude Delarue explains this silence as a way in which we hear our individual music--the timbre of our real voice, the rhythm of our living life, the music that does not live by memory or vanished emotions, the music that must have the art of silence.[9] The opposition of noise and music with spaces of silence is necessary for balance. This is the pattern in concert music when a composition develops in movements, with each player listening silently at certain times to others, knowing that he will perform when the time comes.

It is the same for our patients during group improvisation. The most difficult task for them is to keep from playing and listen carefully while another expresses himself. The creativity of the ensemble emerges only after everyone in the group has listened to the other participants. If music is the support of movement expression, then silence can also play the very same role. As Marcel Marceau once put it during a television interview, "Silence is the mime's music."[10]

During an interview in August 1981, Jean-Louis Barrault united the concepts of life, rhythm, music, and silence into a formula that allows the whole being to participate. He said that one must enter music as if bathed in it. Music is made of silence and silence of music. When one finally awakens to that consciousness of silence and the silence of music, then one becomes connected to music.

---

[9]Claude Delarue, *Vivre la musique* (Paris: Tchou, 1978), p. 87.

[10]Interview with Marcel Marceau, French television network, July 1975.

Some silences are filled with sense and music; others are distressing, empty, synonymous with loneliness and lack of communication. Perhaps intensely experienced music will help dispel these negative feelings.

The Body: A Vehicle for Listening and Expression

Interpretation

Music and movement, inseparable, join together during the interpreter's performance. Sound becomes a mode for bodily expression. Musical and motoric activity emerge from this union. The artist perceives his instrument as an extension of his body. The violinist is not merely making the instrument vibrate with his fingers; his whole being intervenes, tense and vibrating, ready to create sound.

The conductor uses the baton as an intermediate object that clarifies the gesture and extends it without need of words. The union between body and music is even closer in vocal music, a prolongation of breathing, causing a very deep emotional resonance to be induced. G. Rosolato wrote in 1969 that the voice, as an emanation, a corporal aura, can be considered as an intermediate object that goes back through myth and fantasy to that "self" which sorts out these inner voices and, through them, goes back to the "that" of expression.[11]

Listening to Music

Listening is essentially an active rather than a passive step. Music penetrates deeply into the listener who "lives it" within his body. The music coming from outside meets our inner music. This "setting into resonance" is the very condition for listening and will become the primary condition for therapeutic listening. It sets the stage for the exchange between music and the listener. The affective resonance of a musical work is the result of putting the sonorous object into relation with the elements of the subject's personality, his interests, his desires, and his needs. Listening is never passive. It is by nature an everlasting movement. Rosolato tells us that sounds passively heard link up with a prior song that is prepared to take shape by means of memories and that finds its voice in a synergistic balance between

---

[11]G. Rosolato, *Essais sur le symbolisme* (Paris: Gallimard, 1969), p. 210.

the external and internal.[12] The metaphor works well, provided the adverb "passively" is eliminated, since listening cannot be passive.

The sonorous waves reach not only our ears but the whole surface of our bodies and can even generate movement. In certain cultures, the spontaneous reaction toward music through movement is something natural. Examples of this can be found in jazz and also African and Balinese music. Our culture, however, allows us only one acceptable way to listen to music, and that is to keep still. We regard this as the way to become educated by the experience.

The young child, on the other hand, spontaneously reacts to music by moving. As he matures, however, he is taught to stifle this spontaneity, although he remains, for some time, able to express the effects of listening through a glance, facial expressions, sounds he utters, and movements-- aspects of a game described by D. W. Winnicott.[13]

Zoltan Kodaly's educational approach is an attempt to help the child rediscover this spontaneity. The relationship between the child and the music is formed by means of movement. This body expression, lost to the adult, can be rediscovered as a way of expression and communication that is ultimately useful in human relations. The bodily experience of the music suggests strongly that music can be a support in techniques for rehabilitation of bodily functions.

Improvisation and Creativity

The point of music is to develop listening aptitude and the ability to express oneself through sounds. The ear, the voice, and the whole body are involved. Instrumental playing allows movement and breathing to act as mediators in the relationship between the performer and the sonorous object. Instruments extend the body and permit expression and communication without need of words. The creative action results in the creation of the sonorous object. The amateur about to improvise experiences the created music as a unique way of self-expression, at once very close to the body and the vibrations set in motion. The music that pours forth may be an elaborate composition written according to the

---

[12]Ibid., p. 257.

[13]D. W. Winnicott, *Jeu et Réalité* (Paris: Gallimard, 1976).

rules. The non-musician, however, may experience improvisation on the simplest level. The goal is not to produce a great work of art but to induce the emotional expression and communication made possible by the creative experience.

The creative act engenders the notions of delight and pleasure. We are situated in the potential space of which Winnicott speaks, a place and time where everything can be played and played again through the creative energy that is mobilized.[14]

The idea of using music as a cure, to deepen and induce body expression with a therapeutic aim in mind, is still regarded with skepticism. The approach may indeed be useful for some patients and not for others. Music Therapy unites the psychical fact, the listening, and everything it generates, as well as the materialization of the psychical fact in the musical act through improvising and interpretation. The musical phenomenon is at once sonorous vibration felt inside the body, a source of energy, and semantic content insofar as it is information.

The conclusion is best expressed by Pierre Schaeffer's synthetical concept of music. For him, music is a globalizing activity, it is to think with the hands, to prepare sources in order to create objects, and to prepare relations in order to create structures.[15]

---

[14]Ibid., p. 15.

[15]Pierre Schaeffer, *Traité des objets musicaux* (Paris: Seuil, 1966), p. 185.

REFERENCES

Ansermet, Ernest. *Les fondements de la musique dans la conscience humaine.* 2 vols. Neuchatel: La Baconnière, 1961.

Blacking, J. *How Musical Is Man?* London: Faber & Faber, 1976.

Chailley, J. "Essai sur les structures mélodiques." *Revue de Musicologie* 44 (1959):139-75.

Delarue, Claude. *Vivre la musique.* Paris: Tchou, 1978.

Matras, J. J. *Le son.* Paris: Que sais-je? P.U.F., 1967.

Porte, D. *Science de la musique.* Paris: Bordas, 1977.

Rosolato, G. *Essais sur le symbolisme.* Paris: Gallimard, 1969.

Schaeffer, Pierre. *Traité des objets musicaux.* Paris: Seuil, 1966.

Verdeau-Paillès, Jacqueline. *La musique et l'expression corporelle en thérapeutique psychiatrique.* Paris: Masson, 1982.

Winnicott, D. W. *Jeu et Réalité.* Paris: Gallimard, 1976.

MUSIC IN OPERANT PROCEDURES FOR
THE COMATOSE PATIENT

by

MARY ELINOR BOYLE

This paper presents material supplementary to the research initially conducted by Boyle and Greer (1983).

This study sought to address the question of whether the use of music as a contingent reinforcer would increase the frequency of specified motor behaviors of vegetative comatose patients to verbal experimental directions. Three single subject experiments were conducted. Each experiment employed a multiple baseline design across three patient behaviors. The behaviors examined varied according to the capabilities of each patient. These included lateral head movement, mouth movement, eye focus, and eye blinking. The treatment of contingent music consisted of 15-sec segments of preferred music following emission of a correct response. The selection of preferred music was determined by conversation with family members. The baselines of behaviors of each patient showed stable patterns with minimal or no responses. However, 15-sec of contingent music for each correct response produced spiking patterns in the data. These spiking patterns, present during the contingent music phase for all patients, showed the patients to be unresponsive at times and quite responsive at other times. Notable increases in the number of correct responses for all three behaviors were found in Patient 1. Increases in responses for two of the three dependent variables were observed for Patients 2 and 3. For Patient 3, a declining trend in all responses became evident near the conclusion of the experiment. He died within one week of termination of the procedures. The magnitude of the differences may be related to the complexity of the behaviors required and the health of the patients as well as the reinforcing properties of the music.

For many, coma is a transitory phase to either death or recovery. For others, the *persistent vegetative state* (Jennett & Plum, 1972) is an enduring nightmare. The transient quality of coma belies its permanent consequences for these victims. Despite its consequences, "coma remains one of the most enigmatic and least predictable conditions in clinical medicine" (de la Torre, Trimble, Beard, Hanlon, & Surgeon, 1978, p. 304). This situation persists notwithstanding technological advances in medical care, including computerized transaxial tomography, spectral analysis of electroencephalography, and comatosensory evoked potentials measurements. De la Torre et al. (1978) question "whether at any time or under certain circumstances, e.g., appropriate therapy, a 'negative recovery' potential is capable of reversing to a 'positive recovery' pattern" (p. 316). They have pioneered the use of somatosensory evoked potentials measurements to predict recovery or nonrecovery of patients from coma. "Recovery" from coma here refers to any condition varying from no impairment to severe impairment, and "nonrecovery" refers to "death or vegetative coma" (p. 305). This question confronts not only researchers but those caring for comatose patients. With the extraordinary medical procedures now available to patients, under what conditions is it in the patient's best interest to prolong his/her life?

Before these questions can be answered, serious investigations relating to "quality of life" issues must be undertaken. The investigations to the present time have primarily involved either diagnosis or predicted outcome data following hospital admission and surgical procedures. The effect(s) the variable of learning may generate for patients in vegetative or awakening states following comas has not been investigated. Because neuropsychology and neurophysiology are still in the embryonic eras, constructs such as neuronal plasticity and alternative neural pathways are as yet unknown factors affecting consideration of these issues.

The technology of a burgeoning new field, behavioral medicine, offers an avenue for investigation and potential treatment of patients awakening from coma. Behavioral medicine is an emerging field employing clinical techniques "derived from the experimental analysis of behavior . . . for the evaluation, prevention, management, or treatment of physical disease or physiological dysfunction. . ." (Pomerleau & Brady, 1979, p. xii). It is within this framework that the viability of operant feedback procedures employing music for comatose patients will be addressed. In conducting this preliminary research, the investigator acknowledges the humbling directive of Miller (1980) to researchers in the behavioral spheres: "Fumble around until you find something that works."

Coma

To provide a forum for questions of appropriate diagnosis and treatment of coma and brain death, the New York Academy of Sciences sponsored a 1978 international symposium on brain death, states of consciousness, and coma. Despite this, no one definition of coma was promulgated. However, a widely accepted definition of coma is that proposed by Posner (1978): "those states in which cognitive functions are diminished and the patient is unresponsive to all outside stimuli" (p. 218).

The Vegetative State

The term, the *persistent vegetative state,* was first used by Jennett and Plum in 1972 to denote a state in which "the essential component . . . is the absence of any adaptive response to the external environment, the absence of any evidence of a functioning mind which is either receiving or projecting information, in a patient who has long periods of wakefulness" (p. 736). Other terms used to describe this population or subsets of it include: comavigil, the apallic syndrome, cerebral death, and neocortical death (Korein, 1978; Plum & Posner, 1980). Although some authors regard the vegetative state as a form of coma, the more common interpretation allows for a more conservative estimate of coma as a sleeplike state where the patient is unarousable to external stimuli (Plum & Posner, 1980).

Standardized procedures have been developed for testing responsiveness of the comatose patient to external stimuli. The Glasgow Coma Scale examines the best eye-opening, verbal, and motor responses occurring in given time periods (Habbema, Braakman, & Avezaat, 1979; Teasdale, Murray, Parker, & Jennett, 1979). The Munich Coma Scale uses additive scales to rate susceptibility to stimulation and reactivity (Brinkmann, von Cramon, & Schulz, 1976). Stimulation involves electrical, tactile, acoustic, and optic devices, and reactions are motoric, mimic, orientating, or communicative responses. These standardized scales are not widely used, nor do they measure operant responses. The studies reported here were designed to apply the technology of the experimental analysis of behavior to test the responsiveness of comatose patients.

There are several studies dealing with profoundly retarded individuals who were described as vegetative (Brownfield & Keehn, 1966; Fuller, 1949; Rice & McDaniel, 1966; Rice, McDaniel, Stallings, & Gatz, 1967). Coma patients and profoundly retarded individuals are similar in their lack of responses, but their conditioned reinforcers may be different. Dorow (1975) conditioned music stimuli for retarded individuals until music was as effective as food for reinforcing responses to verbal commands. Without special reinforcement conditioning procedures, only primary reinforcers are viable for many profoundly retarded individuals. However, the comatose patients have had many conditioned reinforcers prior to trauma. Also, primary reinforcers are often difficult to use with comatose patients because of the mechanized life support systems

51

(e.g., oxygen, gastrostomy tubes, tracheal tubes, and ventilators) and their tentative and often precarious state.

Music was selected as a contingency for the patients reported here because it seemed suited to the limitations of the patients while simultaneously tapping their potential to be controlled by conditioned reinforcers from their own unique histories. There is extensive literature on music as a reinforcer for a wide variety of responses as well as on the variables related to conditionability (Greer, 1981). In addition, music is unobtrusive, easy to administer, unlikely to produce satiation, and unlikely to create resistance from caretakers, medical personnel, or members of the patients' families.

The question addressed in the experiments is: Can operant music procedures be used to assess environmental control of overt responses of comatose patients in a *vegetative state?*

Method

Three patients were selected because of interest by their relatives and physicians.

Patient 1

The patient was a 56-y-o-male Caucasian, comatose as a result of an accident six months prior to the onset of the experiment. He sustained injuries including severe brain stem injury, a left subdural hematoma, right hygroma, and several fractures. At the time of admission to a rehabilitation hospital, the patient was diagnosed as in a vegetative state. He was observed to have spontaneous eye blinking, mouth, and right hand movements. The patient infrequently blinked his eyes and, upon verbal direction to do so, squeezed a hand placed in his right hand.

Patient 2

The patient was a 31-y-o-female Caucasian who had been in a persistent vegetative state for 38 months prior to onset of the experiment. She had severe anoxic brain damage as a result of respiratory arrest, a complication of Guillan Barre Syndrome. The patient sustained injuries including cortical and probable brain stem injury, multiple contractures, a seizure disorder, and spasticity and rigidity of all extremities. Two physicians obtained contradictory pupillary responses to light and corneal responses. Loud noises elicited grimacing and jerking behaviors from her. Ordinarily, her mouth remained closed while moving in a chewing/sucking manner. The tracheostomy site had never completely closed. The patient's eyes rarely focused on any person or object but moved in a continuous, roving pattern.

Patient 3

The patient was a 44-y-o-black Hispanic male. As the result of a cerebral vascular accident ten months prior to onset of the experiment, he was in a semi-comatose state. The patient had brain stem injury, spastic involvement of all extremities, a seizure disorder, and an extremely labile hypertensive condition. Staff members had observed the patient move his head slightly toward family members' voices and open his eyes for them. His right extremities were more spastic than his left extremities. However, in both cases a therapist could, with effort, bring them around to full extension. Bilateral Babinski signs were present. No plantar response was present.

Data Collection

Definitions of Behaviors. The three dependent variables for Patient 1 were: (a) eye blinking movement, (b) finger movements, and (c) mouth movements. Eye blinking movement consisted of definite movements of the eyelids in which the upper and lower eyelids touched one another and then separated. If the movement occurred so rapidly that the experimenter and/or reliability observer were not certain it happened, it was not counted as a definite eye blink. Finger movement consisted of any movement of the fingers. Mouth movement was any movement of the jaw.

The three dependent variables for Patients 2 and 3 were: (a) lateral head movement, (b) eye focus, and (c) mouth opening. Lateral head movement consisted of any head movement to either side. Either a slight tremor sometimes observable or breathing movements were excluded. Eye focus was defined as an interval in which: the patient opened his/her eyes so that both pupils could be seen, and the patient looked at the experimenter's face for two seconds. Mouth opening consisted of the movement of the patient's mandible so that the lips parted and the teeth or tongue were visible.

Procedures. The procedures used were standard direct observation technique involving discrete trial event recording. Responses to verbal commands given at discrete intervals served as the dependent variables. Each session consisted of 11 trials for each of three behaviors per patient. For each session, the first of each set of 11 trials was physically and verbally prompted, and the following 10 were only verbally prompted. One exception to this serial presentation order was made for Patient 1. This involved a randomized probe for Session 119. There were no physically prompted trials during this session. Thirty verbally prompted trials were presented to the patient in a randomized order. Exceptions to the serial presentation order were made for Patients 2 and 3 during the 9th and 10th sessions of each 10-session grouping. For Patients 2 and 3, if he/she had his/her eyes closed for five consecutive trials in which there were no correct responses, during either the serial or randomized trial presentations, the experimenter shook the patient until his/her eyes spontaneously opened.

During baseline, the experimenter activated a recording of a 10-sec observe interval following each verbal direction. At the end of the observe interval, the experimenter or observer activated a stop watch for a period of 25-sec to include a 15-sec intratrial interval of silence and a 10-sec intertrial interval of silence. During the 15-sec intratrial interval, the experimenter and observer recorded whether or not the behavior occurred during the previous observe interval.

Treatment procedures differed from baseline procedures in the contingent application of 15-sec of preferred music following immediately upon performance of the desired behavior. In those trials in which the desired behavior was not performed, a 15-sec interval of silence replaced a 15-sec interval of music. During the first prompted trial in each sequence as treatment was instituted for each dependent variable, 15-sec of preferred music followed the experimenter's physical prompts and verbal directions. During the subsequent 10 unprompted trials, 15-sec of preferred music were contingent upon correct responses to verbal directions of the experimenter. A 10-sec intertrial interval of silence followed music or silence in the treatment condition.

Contingent Music

The manipulated independent variable consisted of the playback to the patient of selected music excerpts contingent upon the patients'correct responses. Immediately upon elicitation of a desired response, the experimenter activated by foot pedal a cassette tape recorder, which then played a 15-sec segment of music. The selection of preferred music was determined by conversation with the patients' families. For Patient 1, the soundtrack from "Camelot" was chosen. For Patient 2, "Linda Ronstadt 1980 Tour" was chosen. For Patient 3, the selections were: "Disfrutelo Hasta el Cabo!" by El Gran Combo de Puerto Rico and "Album Homenaje! 30 Anose do Victor Pinero: Los Melodicos."

Design

A multiple baseline design employing an ABAB withdrawal feature was used.

Reliability

Reliability (interobserver agreement) was taken for 55 of 140 sessions for Patient 1. Three separate reliability estimates were computed. The first was an overall estimate across the three behaviors for both occurrences and nonoccurrences of the behaviors. This resulted in a 97,76% reliability estimate. The second estimate was calculated for each behavior separately for both occurrences and nonoccurrences of the behaviors. This resulted in a 97.45% reliability estimate for eye blinking, a 98.09% estimate for mouth movement, and a 96.38% reliability estimate for finger movement. The third reliability estimate was calculated by behavior, but only for occurrences of the behavior. This resulted in a 90.98% reliability estimate for eye blinking, a 93.85% reliability estimate for mouth movement, and an 89.65% reliability estimate for finger movement.

Reliability was taken for 42 of 79 sessions for Patient 2. The overall estimate across the three behaviors for both occurrences and nonoccurrences was 98.38%. The second estimate was calculated for each behavior separately for both occurrences and nonoc-currences of the behaviors. This resulted in a 95.48% reliability estimate for eye focus, a 99.29% reliability estimate for lateral head movement, and a 100% reliability estimate for mouth opening. The third reliability estimate for occurrences of each behavior resulted in an 80.76% reliability estimate for eye focus, a 97.47% reliability estimate for lateral head movement, and a 100% reliability estimate for mouth opening.

Reliability was taken for 31 of the 65 sessions for Patient 3. The three reliability estimates calculated employed the same formulas as with Patients 1 and 2. The first estimate for all three behaviors across occurrences and nonoccurrences was 98.45%. The second reliability estimate for each behavior separately by occurrences and nonoccurrences was 98.44% for eye focus, 96.56% for lateral head movement, and 99.69% for mouth opening. The third reliability estimate for occurrences only resulted in a 74.43% reliability estimate for eye focus, 65.75% reliability estimate for lateral head movement, and an 89% reliability estimate for mouth opening.

Results

The results are shown in Figures 1, 2, and 3. Patient 3 died one week following termination of the experiment.

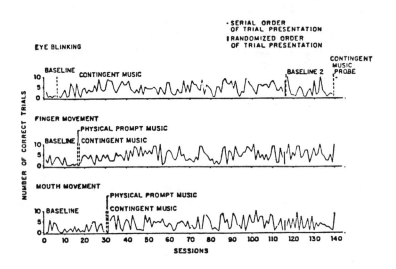

Figure 1. Successfully Completed Trials per Session for Eye Blinking, Finger Movements, and Mouth Movements for Patient 1.

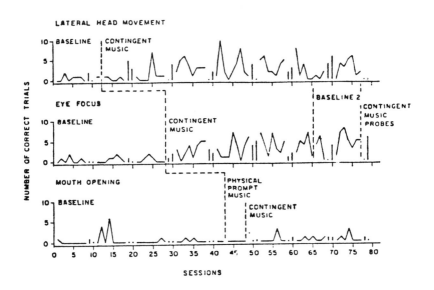

Figure 2. Successfully Completed Trials per Session for Lateral Head Movement, Eye Focus, and Mouth Opening for Patient 2.

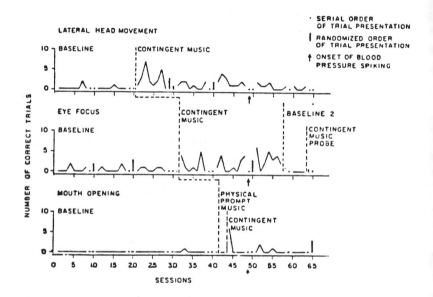

Figure 3. Successfully Completed Trials per Session for Lateral Head Movement, Eye Focus, and Mouth Opening for Patient 3.

REFERENCES

Boyle, M. E., & Greer, R. D. (1983). Operant procedures and the comatose patient. *Journal of Applied Behavior Analysis, 16(1),* 3-12.

Brinkmann, R., von Cramon, D., & Schulz, H. (1976). The Munich coma scale (MCS). *Journal of Neurology, Neurosurgery, and Psychiatry, 39,* 788-793.

Brownfield, E. D., & Keehn, J. D. (1966). Operant conditioning in Trisomy-18. *Journal of Abnormal Psychology, 71,* 413-415.

de la Torre, J. C., Trimble, J. L., Beard, R. T., Hanlon, K., & Surgeon, J. W. (1978). Comatosensory evoked potentials for the prognosis of coma in humans. *Experimental Neurology, 60,* 304-317.

Dorow, L. G. (1975). Conditioning music and approval as new reinforcers for imitative behavior with the severely retarded. *Journal of Music Therapy, 12,* 33-39.

Fuller, P. R. (1949). Operant conditioning of a vegetative human organism. *American Journal of Psychology, 62,* 587-590.

Greer, R. D. (1981). An operant approach to motivation and affect: Ten years of research in music learning. In *Documentary Report of the National Symposium on the Applications of Psychology to the Teaching and Learning of Music,* 102-121. Washington, D.C.: M.E.N.C. Press.

Habbema, J. D. F., Braakman, R., & Avezaat, C. J. J. (1979). Prognosis of the individual patient with severe head injury. *Acta Neurochirurgia, Supp. 28,* 158-160.

Jennett, B., & Plum, F. (1972). Persistent vegetative state after brain damage: A syndrome in search of a name. *Lancet, 1,* 734-737.

Korein, J. (1978). The problem of brain death: Development and history. *Annals of the New York Academy of Science, 315,* 293-306.

Miller, N. E. (1980, December). How the brain affects the health of the body. Address at the *Association for the Advancement of Behavior Therapy Annual Conference,* New York.

Plum, F., & Posner, J. B. (1980). *The diagnosis of stupor and coma.* Philadelphia, Pennsylvania: F. A. Davis Company.

Pomerleau, O. F., & Brady, J. P. (1979). Introduction: The scope and promise of behavioral medicine. In O. F. Pomerleau & J. P. Brady (Eds.), *Behavioral medicine: Theory and practice,* i-xxvi. Baltimore, Maryland: Williams & Wilkins.

Posner, J. B. (1978). Coma and other states of consciousness: The differential diagnosis of brain death. *Annals of the New York Academy of Sciences, 315,* 215-227.

Rice, H. K., & McDaniel, M. W. (1966). Operant behavior in vegetative patients. *The Psychological Record, 16,* 279-281.

Rice, H. K., McDaniel, M. W., Stallings, V. D., & Gatz, M. J. (1967). Operant behavior in vegetative patients 11. *The Psychological Record, 17,* 449-460.

Teasdale, G., Murray, G., Parker, L., & Jennett, B. (1979). Adding up the Glasgow coma score. *Acta Neurochirurgia, Supp. 28,* 13-16.

MUSIC THERAPY IN MEDICAL TECHNOLOGY:
ORGAN TRANSPLANTS

by

ALICIA CLAIR GIBBONS and DAWN L. MCDOUGAL

The information explosion of the 1980s has contributed to the ever-increasing sophistication in medical technology. Along with this technology, medical specialties have continued to develop and have precipitated a segmentalist approach to the treatment of physical illness and disability. Such an approach has tended to depersonalize patient treatment, and patients, with their families, have reacted with growing concern for quality of life.

Generally, physical health is an important component of one's life quality, and there is increasing awareness that emotional and social factors are also critical. The interaction of these factors and their impact on patients can be determined only by the individual patients who are affected by them and who must ultimately judge their worth. It is clear that medical technology can optimize physical functioning, but unless the human responses to physical illness or disability and its treatment are considered, life quality will be judged unsatisfactory and may become even more unsatisfactory with time.

The patients' concern for quality of life has influenced physicians' attitudes about health care and ways in which it is provided. Gelman et al. (1985) report that Dr. William Myerson, Director of Behavioral Sciences at the Sid W. Richardson Institute for Preventive Medicine, has said physicians have begun to recognize the importance of treatment for the whole person. In Myerson's opinion, it is narrow-minded to think illness is related to a single, unitary factor. He believes, instead, that illness is an integration of many factors.

With this change in attitude have come attempts to move from the segmentalist approach to an integrated team effort in patient care. Such attempts have led to incorporating psychiatrists, psychologists, and social workers on medical teams in efforts to treat the whole person. Dr. Clive Callendar, a transplant surgeon at Howard University Hospital, has been involved in a weekly counseling group for kidney transplant patients. In a joint report (Callendar et al., 1980, p. 86), he stated:

> The prime objective of the transplant surgeon
> is to restore the quality of life that existed
> before renal disease occurred. Transplantation

61

alone is often unsuccessful in achieving this objective. The realization of this prompted me to get involved with the group approach to the medical, social, and rehabilitative needs of the renal patient.

Favorable changes in patient recovery and satisfaction with the "whole patient" treatment concept are also substantiated by Simonton, Matthews-Simonton, and Creighton (1978). Their work has directed attention to success through innovative treatment modes. Such success may stimulate additional innovations that may incorporate other disciplines including the creative arts therapies.

The purpose of this paper is to develop a rationale for the use of music therapy in the care of kidney, liver, and bone marrow transplant recipients, donors, and their families. Of particular concern are the emotional responses and social adjustments associated with prognosis, pain, and the highly technical medical procedures after which quality of life is generally measured in terms of physical parameters.

The potential impact of music therapy on the transplant process must begin with a discussion of the characteristics associated with: (a) the pretransplant, (b) the immediate posttransplant, and (c) the later posttransplant stages.

In the pretransplant stage, many patients have unrealistic expectations for recovery following surgery. Patients often conceptualize their poorly functioning organ as a broken automobile part that, upon replacement, allows the system to run smoothly again. Unfortunately, the immunological system cannot accept new parts easily, and patients must be made aware they may never recover the physical functioning levels experienced before illness.

It is extremely important that patients realize the risks of transplant surgery and the prognosis for survival. The risk and survival rates vary with each procedure, and kidney transplant patients generally have the greatest probability for survival. According to Arehart-Treichel (1983), patients who receive live kidneys from relatives have a one year survival rate of 97%, while those who receive cadaver kidneys have a rate of 90%. The one year survival rate for liver transplant patients is slightly less at 79%, while bone marrow patients have the lowest survival rate, a mere 30% (Brown & Kelly, 1976). Because of the risk and the probabilities for survival, patients may choose other treatment methods such as dialysis or chemotherapy.

Aside from risk and survival factors, the most important issue for consideration in the decision to undergo transplantation is postsurgery quality of life. Researchers have examined three parameters in their attempts to describe life quality after transplantation: physical well-being, emotional well-being, and social well-being. Simmons and Kamstra (1980) interviewed 148 transplant patients at four points in time: shortly before transplant, three weeks posttransplant, one year posttransplant, and five to nine years posttransplant. Results indicated physical well-being one year following surgery had increased while difficulty with daily activities decreased significantly. However, five to nine years posttransplant, some difficulties with daily activities still persisted. An overall physical health assessment revealed that 32% of the nondiabetic patients were in excellent health, 50% were rated moderately good with some significant physical complaints, 8% were in poor condition, while 10% experienced chronic rejection. The evaluation of diabetic patients' health was worse. None were in excellent condition, 56% were in moderately good condition, and 44% were in poor condition.

Emotional well-being measurements for both diabetic and nondiabetic patients showed increases in self-esteem, independence, and control over destiny, while feelings of depression, self-preoccupation, and anxiety decreased. Social well-being, as measured by the patients' satisfaction with major life roles, indicated more satisfaction after surgery than before, for both nondiabetic and diabetic patients.

These studies indicate quality of life based on measures of physical, emotional, and social well-being increase significantly from pre- to posttransplant stage. However, this does not guarantee a quality of life comparable to that prior to illness. Patients must be made aware of this fact in order to develop realistic expectations and make appropriate decisions concerning transplantation.

Patients may resist efforts to confront them with information concerning the transplant procedures and the prognosis. Brown and Kelly (1976) describe one method that forces bone marrow transplant patients to acknowledge potential risks prior to surgery. This method requires the patient to read and sign a consent form that details the treatment procedures, the 30% survival rate, and the psychological implications of the painful treatment process. Even with this procedure, patients may avoid confronting the frightening issue of death, pain, or sterility, and may often tend to focus on less threatening issues such as hair loss or technical aspects of the procedure.

Once the decision is made to proceed with transplantation, the patient may suffer anxiety related to donor availability. Usually a patient's relative is the preferred donor in kidney and bone marrow transplants, since a related donor increases the probability of graft acceptance. This fact may contribute to high stress levels in the patient's family and may amplify previous family conflicts. When family members are physically matched and judged compatible, they may decide to become donors out of guilt feelings or pressure from their families. Psychiatric evaluation or counseling is recommended for the patient, the potential donor, and the family before the donor is determined.

Psychiatric disturbances in both the donor and the recipient are reported commonly in case study literature. The incidence was also revealed in a survey of liver transplant patients where House, Dubovsky, and Penn (1983) found 95% of preoperative and 100% of postoperative adult transplant patients experienced significant psychiatric distress. House further reported lower figures for kidney transplant patients with 17% of the preoperative patients and 32% of the postoperative patients experiencing psychiatric disturbances. These disturbances included: marked regressive behavior, uncontrolled anger, depression, anxiety, and refusal to cooperate. In addition, 70% of the liver transplant patients suffered from preoperative organic brain syndrome.

The patients' psychiatric disturbances may be exacerbated by procedures specific to each type of transplant. These procedures are particularly difficult for bone marrow patients who are required to spend up to six days in isolation for preparatory immunosuppression treatments. The sterile environment of the isolation unit during this time often results in feelings of loneliness, barriers to closeness and touching, sensory deprivation, and much unstructured time in which to contemplate possible death. As a result, the bone marrow patient has intense emotional needs, and psychiatric disturbances are probable. These disturbances make recovery from surgery even more difficult.

The early period following surgery is called the immediate posttransplant stage. When it is free of medical complications, the recipient feels euphoric and thankful. However, the first sign of possible transplant rejection results in intense anxiety. To describe their fears of transplant rejection, patients report feelings of "sitting on a powder keg" (Freyberger, 1983). During this time, patients may alternate between periods of agitation and depression. Uncontrolled anger at the medical staff usually results in additional pain from the treatments delivered.

Once the rejection crisis passes, the patient often experiences difficulty in conceptually integrating the new organ. One case report describes a patient who complained of what he called the "Frankenstein Syndrome," in which he likened himself to a freakish creation (House et al., 1983). Stewart (1983) reports that the new organ is often seen as part of him- or herself. If and when the internalization process occurs, the recipient may assume behavioral characteristics of the donor (Jacobs & Viederman, 1982).

In addition to emotional reactions associated with organ integration, the patient has feelings about the donor. When the donor is a relative, the patient may experience feelings of guilt and indebtedness. The donor, on the other hand, may want an expression of gratitude from the recipient. He or she may also feel ignored by the family, as the family's attention is focused primarily on whether the graft will be accepted. If the organ is rejected, both the donor and the recipient feel a deep sense of loss, depression, guilt, and hopelessness. The recipient feels further anxiety about the possibility of death, the probability of another life support process such as dialysis, and/or the chance of another transplant surgery. If these feelings are not communicated and resolved, family conflicts may escalate to monumental proportions.

When the transplant is successful, the patient moves into the later posttransplant stage where he must cope with the realities of a drug- and diet-regulated life to prevent future rejection. Immunosuppressant drugs such as Prednisone and Imuran may cause unpleasant side effects. These side effects may include: decreased resistance to infection, variable degree of cushinoid appearance (puffy facial features and abdominal bulge), and mood swings between mania and depression (Fortner-Frazier, 1981). The patient will be forever faced with meeting the rising costs of medication, the regular extensive medical checkups, and the reality of medical dependence for life.

In this stage, socialization is resumed but may be particularly difficult. Support groups and social contacts are often lost during the long period of hospitalization, and the patient may find it extremely difficult to move into social relationships. In addition, vocational rehabilitation may be difficult. Some patients cannot meet the physical requirements of their previous jobs, must reevaluate their vocational skills, and move into new areas of employment. The patient is faced with the additional stresses associated with changes in his work while dealing with his fragile health.

In summary, the literature delineates several emotional and social factors that are stressors accompanying transplantation.

65

These include: fear; anxiety; and depression associated with probable surgical risks, possible rejection, and prognosis; sensory deprivation in the sterile hospital environment; guilt and indebtedness to the donors; physical pain in recovery; difficulty in establishing and re-establishing social relationships; lack of personal control in drug- and diet-regulated life; and loss of self-esteem when physical limitations force employment changes. These factors severely stress patients and their families, often to the point of crisis, as they move through the transplantation process and attempt to pursue and maintain a satisfactory quality in their lives.

Such life quality may be enhanced by music therapy programs. Music may be particularly feasible in therapeutic processes because of its flexibility to meet needs at various physiological, social, and psychological response levels, and because of its pervasiveness in peoples' lives. It is incorporated into the rituals associated with crises and milestones throughout the life cycle, yet it is absent in the crises associated with life-threatening illness and recovery.

Gaston (1968) articulated eight fundamental considerations regarding the use of music in therapy that make it viable in the treatment of the "whole" person: (a) All persons have a need for aesthetic experience; (b) Cultural and social context determine the mode of music expression; (c) Music has the power to draw people together for a common purpose; (d) Music is a form of communication; (e) Music is derived from the emotions; (f) Music is structured reality; (g) Music is a source of gratification; and (h) The potency of music is greatest in the group.

1. All people have a need for aesthetic experience. Music is a form of aesthetic experience that provides sensory and cognitive stimulation in a hospital where such activity is often restricted by a sterile environment.

2. Cultural and social context determine the mode of music expression. As people learn to respond to music, their culture determines not only the appropriate responses but the music that elicits it. Music can, therefore, serve to stimulate particular desired responses in patients.

3. Music has the power to draw people together for a common purpose. The structure and cultural context of music make it possible for the patient to have closeness with family members while in the hospital. This can decrease feelings of isolation and provide opportunities for mutual support.

4. Music is a form of communication. Though not a universal language, due to its cultural context, music still provides the means to communicate emotions in acceptable ways within a particular cultural context. It provides a unique means of communication not

otherwise available, and most people are generally responsive to it. Music, used in a structured therapy session, can facilitate and/or provide the communication desperately needed between transplant recipients, donors, their families, and medical staff.

5. Music is derived from the emotions. It can be used to evoke and enhance positive, threatening, or painful feelings in socially appropriate ways. The diagnosis of serious illness can lead to new patterns of emotional expression that may increase stress in the family. Music may facilitate expression of emotions with as little threat as possible.

6. Music is structured reality. It has order and predictability that make it stable and comfortable. It may contribute greatly to patients' comfort levels in the sterile hospital environment. Using music in structured ways may give patients opportunities for personal control that they are forced to sacrifice in the treatment process. It may also offer opportunities to structure time in the pre- and postsurgery stages and in the lengthy and painful recovery period that follows.

7. Music is a source of gratification. Simonton, Matthews-Simonton, and Creighton (1978) have indicated participation in pleasurable, gratifying experiences can alleviate pain. In addition, music can provide opportunities for successful experience that leads to improved self-esteem in a context where physical illness may have eroded it.

8. The potency of music is greatest in the group. Here there are opportunities for social interaction and reintegration into social contexts of which the transplant patient and his family are deprived. The peer group serves as a referent for appropriate social behaviors and provides much needed support and encouragement. Music can be a significant facilitator in the enhancement of social interactions and of developing relationships.

The literature concerning the physiological influences of music has shown changes in various physiological parameters. Sears (1951) found stimulative music elicited postural tension and sedative music relaxed it. Likewise, stimulative and sedative music can tense or relax muscles (Sears, 1959). Research studies (Michel, 1952; Schrift, 1974; Taylor, 1970) found that music affected the galvanic skin response (GSR). Taylor (1970) concluded that the stimulative or sedative attributes of the music alone are not the sole determinants of its effects, but previous musical experience is also important. Other factors such as personality and preference may also impact the GSR (Ries, 1969).

In addition to GSR, DeJong, Van Mourick, and Schellekens (1973) studied the effects of music on respiration and heart rate. Their findings indicated highly significant changes. Rates were faster with "fast" tempo music and slower with "slow or medium" tempo music. Yet other researchers' findings indicated no significant changes (Ellis & Brighouse, 1972; Zinny & Weidenfeller, 1963; Ruiz, 1979; Malcom, 1981). In a small subject study, Brady, Luborsky, and Kron (1974) reduced blood pressure significantly by means of metronomic clicks as a sound stimulus. Later, Hoffman (1980) studied the effects of music in relaxation training on essentially hypertensive patients. Their hypertension was reduced significantly, and medication dosages were decreased for some.

Some recent observations reveal a possibility for pain control with music when used as a distractor or when combined with relaxation techniques or mental imagery. Empirical evidence to support these observations may prove the efficacy of music in procedures for non-pharmacological pain control.

Evidence for social influences of music suggests musical preferences are socially controlled and influenced by familiarity (Schuessler, 1948). Music is also used to control behavior in the environment through commercial industries such as Muzak (Muzak Corporation, 1974). While Muzak claims to enhance the work environment to promote productivity, other commercial companies use music to cue various situations and the appropriate behavior associated with them, i.e., music that cues the beginning of a ceremony, the opening of a sports event, or the feelings associated with a movie scene.

Because music can be used in social control, it may be used to structure predictable and stable environments for patients and their families who are under stress produced by trauma. A reduction in such stress could result in improved comfort levels; may serve to distract attention from the trauma, thereby reducing its impact; and may subsequently impact the probability for recovery.

In consideration of the psychological influences of music, several researchers have attempted to measure the effect of music on mood. These studies suggest that the existing mood of the listener likely affects his/her emotional response to it (Eagle, 1971). There is also indication that a mood can be altered when music is matched to it and then is gradually changed (Shatin, 1970). Furthermore, there is indication that persons with similar moods respond similarly to the same music (Sopchak, 1955).

Some studies show music affects anxiety as measured by physiological responses and verbal reports. Greenberg and Fisher (1966, 1972) found exciting music produced more anxiety and aggression than calm music. Jellison (1975) found no difference in verbal anxiety reports during calm and exciting music conditions, but subjects in these music conditions reported significantly less anxiety than subjects in a white noise condition.

In other research concerning psychological responses, Ridgeway (1976) found that music aided in dealing with interpersonal interactions; Allen and White (1966) found music a psychotherapeutic agent for improving self-concept; and Heher, Wallach, and Greenberg (1960) found music stimulated arousal. In later work, researchers studied the effect of music therapy sessions on depression, and the effect of music with mental imagery on self-esteem in elderly subjects (Ramsay, 1982; Ice, 1984). Results were not statistically significant, but these findings may have been different with extended treatment conditions over longer periods of time.

The research indicates that music influences physiological, social, and psychological responses to music. While these aspects require further investigation, there is evidence that music has impact. Concomitantly, it can influence treatment in the therapeutic context. The implication is that music therapy may be programmed to impact the emotional and social factors associated with organ transplantation, which may, in turn, affect the anticipatory and recovery processes for patients and their families. Music therapy may be a viable addition to the medical treatment team concerned with quality care delivery, facilitated recovery, and the patients' and the families' satisfaction with the process.

REFERENCES

Allen, W. R., & White, W. F. (1966). Psychodramatic: Affects of music as a psychotherapeutic agent. *Journal of Music Therapy, 3,* 69-71.

Arehart-Treichel, J. (1983, November 19). The organ transplant odyssey. *Science News,* pp. 218-19.

Brady, J. P., Luborsky, L., & Kron, R. (1974). Metronome conditioned relaxation. *Behavior Therapy, 5,* 203-209.

Brown, H. N., & Kelly, M. J. (1976, November-December). Stages of bone marrow transplantation: a psychiatric perspective. *Psychosomatic Medicine, 38,* 441.

Callendar, C. O., Silverman, A., Rice, B., & Green, G. (Summer 1980). Kidney transplantation: its enhancement by a rehabilitation centered counseling group. *Journal of Applied Rehabilitation Counseling, 11,* 85-89.

DeJong, M. A., Van Mourick, K. R., & Schellekens, H. M. (1973). A physiological approach to aesthetic preference. *Psychotherapy and Psychosomatics, 22,* 46-51.

Eagle, C. T., Jr. (1971). *Effects of existing mood and order of presentation of vocal and instrumental music on rated mood responses to that music.* Unpublished doctoral dissertation, University of Kansas, Lawrence.

Ellis, D. S., & Brighouse, G. (1952). Effects of music on respiration and heart rate. *American Journal of Psychology, 65,* 39-47.

Fisher, S., & Greenberg, R. P. (1972). Selective effects upon women of exciting and calm music. *Perceptual and Motor Skills, 34,* 987-990.

Fortner-Frazier, C. L. (1981). *Social Work and Dialysis* (p. 107). Los Angeles: University of California Press.

Freyberger, H. (1983). The renal transplant patient: three-stage model and psychotherapeutic strategies. In N. B. Levy (Ed.), *Psychonephrology 2* (p. 260). New York: Plenum Publishing.

Gaston, E. T. (1968). Man and music. In E. T. Gaston (Ed.), *Music in Therapy* (pp. 21-27). New York: Macmillan Publishing.

Gelman, D., Shapiro, D., Morris, H., Shirley, D., Karagianis, E., & Katz, S. (1985). Patient, heal thyself. *Newsweek, 12,* pp. 82-84.

Greenberg, R. P., & Fisher, S. (1966). Some differential effects of music on projective and structured psychological tests. *Psychological Reports, 28,* 817-20.

Hoffman, J. (1980). *Management of essential hypertension through relaxation training with sound.* Unpublished master's thesis, University of Kansas, Lawrence.

House, R., Dubovsky, S. L., & Penn, I. (1983, August). Psychiatric aspects of hepatic transplantation. *Transplantation, 36,* 149.

Ice, D. (1984). *The effects of music and guided imagery on self-esteem of elderly female care home residents.* Unpublished master's thesis, University of Kansas, Lawrence.

Jacobs, A. R., & Viederman, M. (1982). Adaptation to kidney transplantation: a case presentation and discussion. *General Hospital Psychiatry, 4,* 302.

Jellison, J. A. (1975). The effect of music on autonomic stress responses and verbal reports. In C. K. Madsen, R. Greer, & C. H. Madsen (Eds.) *Research in Music Behavior* (pp. 206-219). New York: Teachers College Press.

Malcom, G. L. (1981). *Effect of rhythm on heart rate of musicians.* Unpublished master's thesis, University of Kansas, Lawrence.

Michel, D. E. (1952). *Effects of stimulative and sedative music on respiration and psychogalvanic reflex as observed in seventh grade students.* Unpublished research paper, University of Kansas, Lawrence.

Muzak Corporation (1974). *Significant Studies of the effects of Muzak on employee performance.* New York: Muzak Corporation.

Ramsay, D. (1982). *Music therapy and depression in the elderly.* Unpublished master's thesis, University of Kansas, Lawrence.

Ridgeway, C. L. (1976). Affective interaction as a determinant of musical involvement. *The Sociological Quarterly, 17,* 414-28.

Ries, H. A. (1969). GSR and breathing aptitude related to emotional reactions to music. *Psychonomic Science, 14,* 62-64.

Ruiz, O. M. (1979). *Effect of music on heart rate.* Unpublished master's thesis, University of Kansas, Lawrence.

Schuessler, K. F. (1948). Social background and musical taste. *American Sociological Review, 13,* 330-35.

Sears, W. W. (1959). *A study of some effects of music upon muscle tension as evidence by electromyographic recordings.* Unpublished doctoral dissertation, University of Kansas, Lawrence.

Sears, W. W. (1951). *Postural response to recorded music.* Unpublished master's thesis, University of Kansas, Lawrence.

Shatin, L. (1970). Alteration of mood via music: a study of the vectoring effect. *Journal of Psychology, 75,* 81-86.

Shrift, D. C. (1974). *The galvanic skin response to two contrasting types of music.* Unpublished master's thesis, University of Kansas, Lawrence.

Simmons, R. G., & Kamstra, L. (1980). Long-term rehabilitation of transplant patients. *Proceedings of Clinical Dialysis and Transplantation, 10,* 43.

Simonton, O. C., Matthews-Simonton, S., & Creighton, J. L. (1978). *Getting well again.* (chap. 7). New York: Bantam Books.

Sopchak, A. L. (1955). Individual differences in responses to music. *Psychology Monograph, 69,* 1-20.

Stewart, R. S. (1983). Psychiatric issues in renal dialysis and transplantation. *Hospital and Community Psychiatry, 34,* 624.

Taylor, D. B. (1970). *Subject responses to precategorized stimulative and sedative music.* Unpublished master's thesis, University of Kansas, Lawrence.

Wallach, M. A., & Greenberg, C. (1960). Personality functions of symbolic sexual arousal to music. *Psychology Monograph, 74,* 1-18.

Zinny, G. H., & Weidenfeller, E. W. (1963). Effects of music upon GSR and heartrate. *American Journal of Psychology, 76,* 311-14.

UTILIZING MUSIC AS A TOOL FOR HEALING

by

ARTHUR W. HARVEY

Since antiquity, the relationship between music and medicine has been an important one. Publications in the fields of medicine, philosophy, religion, anthropology, musicology, music therapy, psychology, and other health-related professions have sought to present a rationale for the interrelationship of music and medicine. Many of the periodicals and reports focus on a historical precedent for the use of music in medicine. *Music and Medicine,* by Schullian and Schoen (1948) was the first of recent books to offer a broad overview of this topic. A more extensive research study into the correlation between medicine and music, *Musik und Medizin,* was written by Werner Kuemmel (1977). The English translation of the title and subtitle reads: Music and Medicine: Their Interrelationship in Theory and Practice from 800-1800. The next account appeared in the *Journal of Music Therapy* in an article by Dale Taylor (1981) entitled: "Music in General Hospital Treatment from 1900-1950." At the Third International Symposium on Music in Medicine, Education, and Therapy for the Handicapped, Rosalie Rebollo Pratt (1985) presented a paper, "The Historical Relationship between Music and Medicine," that reviewed the history of music and medicine and music therapy.

Rather than repeat what was covered in those publications, this paper will focus on a contemporary and specific approach to music and medicine: a proposal that music can be shown to have a direct effect upon both the physiological and psychological functions of the human organism and, as such, can be utilized for both remediative and preventive medicine. It is anticipated that these ideas will be developed and tested more thoroughly through the establishment of a proposed Institutes for the Study of Music, Mind, and Medicine. The rationale for such a concept is predicated upon the following assumptions:

1. The center of control for the human organism is the brain.
2. The field of the neurosciences is currently one of the fastest growing areas of scientific studies.
3. Music is processed by the brain and through the brain, after which it can then affect us in many ways.
4. The field of Psychoneuroimmunology presents a case for the human organism's ability to provide for its own health through hemeostatic regulation of neurotransmitters and hormones. This

process enables the body's own immune system to function in such a way as to produce and to facilitate physical and mental health.

5. Music can have a positive effect upon both neural functions and hormonal activity and, as such, can facilitate the healthy functioning of the body's own immune and regenerative processes.

Although there are isolated instances of studies that suggest a positive relationship between music and its use in remediative and preventive medicine, the proposal is made for a comprehensive "Brain-Model Approach." This idea is conceptualized in the establishment of the Institutes for the Study of Music, Mind, and Medicine by means of the development of a holistic perspective based on a brain analogy. The Institutes would have several divisions.

The Behavioral and Experimental Studies Division would use an analytical, rational approach (similar to the left cerebral hemisphere) studying such areas as:

1. The effect of music on specific neurotransmitters (endorphins).
2. The effect of music on the endocrine system.
3. The correlation between music and immunology.
4. The effect of music on the limbic system.
5. The development of research on music and surgical procedures.
6. Further study on uses of music in hospital settings that include: childbirth, kidney dialysis, burn patients, chemotherapy, chronic pain, heart catheterization, stress manifestations, pre- and post-operative procedures, remediation of aphasia, and audioanesthesia.
7. The effect of music on the corpus callosum.
8. The effect of music upon the functioning of the reticular activating system.
9. The use of music in maintaining responses in comatose patients.
10. The function of music in teaching minimally brain-damaged patients.

The Transpersonal and Existential Division would rely upon more subjective, intuitive approaches (similar to the right cerebral hemisphere), studying such areas as:

1. The role of music in altering consciousness.
2. The effect of music upon brain functions during brain wave states.
3. The impact of music upon stress reduction.

4. The role of music in synaesthesia.
5. The effects of sound-planned environments upon health.
6. Explorations into music and psychic healing.
7. Extensions of the study of music in suggestopedia.
8. Explorations into music as a source of peak experiences.
9. Studies in differences between aesthetic and religious experiences.
10. Studies of the role music might play in psychoneuroimmunological applications.
11. Comparative ethnomusicological studies on an intercultural scope in relation to health and illness.

The Synthesis and Applied Studies Division would serve to provide both a connecting link or bridge (similar to the role of the corpus callosum) between differing psychological philosophical viewpoints and would provide an integrated or holistic channel through which future studies of the application of music to the field of medicine would emerge.

Current evidence of the interest in establishing a more scientific basis for the relationship between the fields of medicine and music may be seen in recent conferences such as the MEH Symposia, as well as those sponsored by the International Society for Music in Medicine. The Second International Symposium: Music in Medicine was held in October 1984 in Luedenscheid, West Germany, under the leadership of Drs. Droh and Spintge, two of the speakers at this symposium. Another such conference, The Biology of Music Making, was held during July 1984 in Denver, Colorado, under the leadership of Dr. Frank Wilson, who is also a speaker at this symposium. A research cruise entitled "First World Congress: Music in Medicine" is planned for October 1985 aboard the "Mediterranean Sky," sailing through the Greek Isles. Still another organization, The International Arts in Medicine Society, has recently been founded in Philadelphia, Pennsylvania. These events and organizations represent a major effort to provide a synergistic approach to the integration of the fields of music and medicine as a complement to the fine work of the existing arts therapy organizations such as the National Association for Music Therapy, the American Association for Music Therapy, and the American Association of Artists-Therapists.

Several recent publications have explored the implications of music and healing. One of these periodicals is *Brain/Mind Bulletin*. The January 21-February 11, 1985 issue contained an article entitled "Music medicine: a new field emerging." The periodical, *Ear: Magazine of New Music* devoted two complete issues (February/March 1981 and November/December 1984) to the subject, "Music and Sound in Healing." Other publications on this topic include: *The Life Energy in Music: Notes on Music and Sound,* volumes 1 and 2 (1981 and 1983), by Dr. John Diamond, one of our symposium speakers and founder of the Institutes for the Enhancement of Life Energy and Creativity, Valley Cottage, New York; *Sound Health: The Music and Sounds That Make Us Whole,* published in 1985 by Steven Halpern, with Louis Savary; "Music That Strikes a Healing Chord," by Gale Malesky, *Prevention,* October 1983; "Music for a Healthy Heart," by Ed Shanahy, *Keyboard Classics* (1984); and "Music Medicine," by Robert Brody, *Omni,* (April 1984).

Studies published in recent issues of professional journals confirm a growing interest in the application of music to remediative medical treatment procedures and programs. The application of music encompasses the full spectrum of developmental stages, from pre-natal through geriatric.

Dr. Thomas Verny (1982) cites studies that indicate that the unborn child listens to musical and non-musical sounds from the twenty-fourth week in utero. Although the noise level in the uterus is about 85 decibels and is sufficient to mask much sound, external sounds about 85 decibels can increase the fetal heartbeat within five seconds, even though the maternal heartbeat remains unchanged. Studies done by audiologists have shown that the unborn child has distinct musical likes and dislikes, and the fetal response indicates musical preferences. Dr. Dominick Purpura, Professor at the Albert Einstein Medical College and Head of the Study Section on the Brain at the National Institutes of Health, puts the start of auditory awareness between the twenty-eighth and thirty-second week in utero.

The use of music during labor and delivery has been reported with increasing frequency within the past decade. A study by Clark, McCorkle, and Williams (1981) at the University of Kansas Medical Center suggests several functions of music in Prepared Childbirth:

1. Music has the potential for becoming an effective attention-focusing stimulus. Earlier studies suggest that attention-focusing not only increases pain tolerance but may totally eliminate pain sensation.
2. Music may serve as a distraction stimulus, a proven method for pain control.
3. Music can evoke a positive emotional tone and serve as a stimulus for a pleasure response.
4. Music has excellent potential for becoming a conditioned stimulus for relaxation. Neuromuscular relaxation is important.
5. Music, in conjunction with or as a stimulus for guided

imagery enables the mother to focus on visual events mentally and find richer meaning in them.

    6.   Music can serve as a structural aid to breathing and can reinforce and support the breathing patterns and rhythms learned in Lamaze childbirth classes.

    Music Therapy-Assisted Labor and Delivery Approach as developed by Clark, McCorkle, and Williams was initiated in Kansas and Missouri and has since been used by music therapists in conjunction with medical staff at hospitals throughout the United States. A follow-up study by Hanser, Larson, and O'Connell (1983) at the University of the Pacific focused on the "audioanalgesic" effect of music to reduce pain through cued rhythmic breathing, assisting the women in relaxing by prompting positive associations with music. The study yielded rather dramatic results since 100% of the mothers in the experimental group displayed fewer pain responses while music was played during labor.

    A clinical study was conducted by Linda Marley (1984) at Miller Children's Hospital in Long Beach, California, to examine the effectiveness of music in decreasing stress behaviors exhibited by hospitalized infants and toddlers. Salk (1981) observed in his article, "Mother's Beat as an Imprinting Stimulus," that children fell asleep better when they heard the sound of seventy-two beats a minute rather than other sounds. A study by Helen Chetta (1981) in Florida involved music as part of a comprehensive preoperative teaching session aimed at informing pediatric patients about events pertaining to surgery. The group of children receiving music therapy just prior to induction of preoperative medication was consistently rated as indicating less anxiety before and during induction of preoperative medication.

    Researchers at Muzak Corporation (Muzak 1) report that music used within a treatment environment indicated positive results. A significant reduction of stress was found among 286 patients in the pre-operative area at Creighton University/St. Joseph's Hospital in Omaha, Nebraska. The results showed that music exerted a measurable and highly consistent reductive effect on systolic and diastolic blood pressure, pulse rate, and respiration rate. In addition, both patients and medical staff members reported less anxiety and a positive effect upon patients' feeling states and stress levels. In another study at Wassaic Developmental Center for the retarded and neurologically impaired in New Jersey (Muzak 2), a 95% reduction in grand mal seizures was reported.

    At Union Hospital in the Bronx, New York, Muzak Muzak 3) was installed in the pre-operative area, operating rooms, and recovery room in order to observe the effect of music on patients. According to physicians at the hospital, the results were favorable in all areas, and a plan to use music in other areas is under discussion.

At St. Joseph's Hospital in Yonkers, New York, Muzak (Muzak 4) provided musical programming for the Intensive Care Unit (ICU). Specific musical preferences included: an emphasis on major modes rather than minor modes; melodies that were tuneful but not sad or somber; music that would not evoke wistful reminiscences about the "good old days;" and music that would be bright but not exciting. The rhythm had to be regular but not predominant, with enough variation to avoid monotony. Variations in loudness were controlled in the music programs to insure that no sudden musical peaks would precipitate a fatal cardiac arrhythmia. While complete results have not been published, preliminary findings indicate that the ICU's recovery rate has been considerably above the statistical prediction.

In a recent study conducted through Eastern Kentucky University to determine the specific effectiveness of passive listening to sedate music to reduce the "state" level of anxiety of family members waiting for the outcome of surgery, Livingwood, Kiser, and Paige (1984) found that music could be used to reduce anxiety. Recommendations included incorporating music in hospital waiting rooms, patient rooms, and the cafeteria. It was further suggested that health professionals learn about the therapuetic uses of music. For the past ten years, the writer has been leading such in-service and pre-service training programs each semester through the College of Allied Health and Nursing of Eastern Kentucky University.

MacClelland (1979) has noted the following benefits resulting from music used in the operating room:

1. Music creates a warmer, more pleasant environment for the patient and the staff.
2. Music provides a diversion, distracting the patient from strange sights and treatments.
3. The patient undergoing regional anesthetic becomes less restless because discomfort from positioning muscle strains is lessened and the time passes more quickly.
4. The use of headsets muffles extraneous noises and may also keep the patient from overhearing inappropriate conversation.
5. Members of the surgical team work in closer harmony because of decreased levels of frustration and fatigue.
6. Appropriate rhythms may stimulate rapid, coordinated movements.

7. The monotony of preparation and cleanup procedures is reduced, contributing to staff morale and efficiency. MacClelland also suggests that, if music is carried over into the recovery period, patients may experience shortened, more pleasant postanesthetic recovery.

Buckingham (1983) reports a study done at the University of Texas M. D. Anderson Hospital and Tumor Institute by Janet Cook, R.N. in which music was introduced to the hyperthermia treatment section. Cook discovered that patients listening to music while undergoing radiation therapy were more relaxed, with measurable reduction in anxiety levels. Based upon the results of her study, Cook feels that music increases a patient's tolerance for treatments and the hospital environment. She also feels that music can be used in other clinical settings to provide a meaningful contact with the outside world for patients in isolation, the protected environment, or in intensive care units.

In a study at the Sloan-Kettering Memorial Cancer Center in New York City, Lucanne Magill Bailey (1983) found (as have many other studies) that music produces physical and emotional changes in hospitalized cancer patients. However, her study showed that live music affects hospitalized cancer patients significantly more than does tape-recorded music of the same material. In a study through ICM West, Helen Bonny (1983) found that programmed taped music in intensive coronary care units did indeed reduce stress for the patient and created an auxilliary treatment approach for the nursing personnel. The results of the study indicated decreased heart rates, greater tolerance for pain and suffering, lessened anxiety and depression in patients, and positive changes in target behaviors pre- to post-music, as reported by nurse evaluators.

Since it is assumed that the reader will become familiar with the wealth of music therapy listerature and medical reports that provide the foundation upon which current and future studies are done, this paper will deal solely with uses of music in medicine from 1980 - 1985. The Rockefeller Foundation (1978) has published a working report, *The Healing Role of the Arts*. In the report, Marvin Gewirtz of Hospital Audiences, Inc., cites several examples of the connection between arts services and medical treatment and then states that " . . . at this point we have found sufficient evidence to justify further intensive research (dealing with the impact of the creative arts on the healing arts)." Indeed, a core of studies is accumulating today that provides both a foundation for further research and an impetus to explore new horizons.

Maleskey (1983) reports that patients at the Kaiser-Permanente Medical Center in Los Angeles have a choice. When in pain, they can either turn on music or turn to prescriptions. Other hospitals using music as part of their treatment program are the University of Massachussetts Medical Center in Worcester; Beth Israel Hospital in Boston; Hahnemann University Hospital in Philadelphia; Walter Reed Army Medical Center; Mount Zion Hospital in San Francisco; the A.R.E. Medical Center in Phoenix; and the Simonton Cancer Research and Counseling Center in Fort Worth/Dallas. The uses of music in many situations vary from hospital to hospital and may include helping couples celebrate the birth of a baby, aiding a child to prepare for heart catheterization, enabling a stroke victim to learn to speak again (Melodic Intonation Therapy was developed at Boston University School of Medicine), and evoking the memories of a lifetime as someone prepares for death.

In the past few years, audio and video programs have been developed that meet the needs of remediative medicine. Bonny (1983) has created a *Music Rx* cassette program for the Institute of Consciousness and Music (ICM). The University of Massachussetts Medical Center Stress-Reduction and Relaxation Department (Kabat-Zinn, n.d.) has produced a fifty-seven minute video tape with Dr. Jon Kabat-Zinn, Director, and Georgia Kelly providing the musical accompaniment. Kelly also has solo audio recordings. Steven Halpern (1985) has tested his music in a variety of remediative and preventive settings. Ralph Hoy (1972) founded and operates a non-profit service organization called Recordings for Recovery.

As the creative art of music gains more credibility with practitioners of the healing arts, a better understanding of the interdisciplinary aspects of the two fields should develop. Although music is primarily an auditory process, the effects of sound vibrations are processed through and responded to by much of the human organism. Sound vibrations are channeled through the ear as well as skin and bone conduction and are processed in the brain stem (reticular activating system), limbic system (thalamus), cerebral cortex (basically the temporal lobes). Neural impulses trigger autonomic nervous system reactions, which in turn produce changes in respiration, pulse rate, blood pressure, muscle tone, brain wave frequency, galvanic skin response, pilomotor reflexes, pupilary reflexes, gastric motility, etc.

Music is sound organized in time through the interrelated elements of rhythm, melody, harmony, form, texture, and timbre. These musical elements produce emotional responses through variations--the creative component--of dynamics, tempo, consonance/ disonance balance, timbre, and sonority. Harvey (1985) found that there were differing biophysical and psychophysical responses resulting from brain functions in response to sound, and that these responses varied according to the type of perceiver/ respondent. The reader who understands a few of these responses may be motivated to study further this most complex and wonderful relationship, i.e., music that can produce health.

In an age of high stress, it is encouraging to note that music can evoke "natural highs" through inducing the release of endorphins, the brain's own endogenous neurotransmitter opiates. Dr. Avram Goldstein (1985), Addiction Research Center, Stanford, used music chosen by experimental subjects to induce "musical thrills." These "thrills" reflect the spreading of electrical activity in some regions of the brain connected to both limbic (emotional center) and autonomic control centers. Goldstein reported that these "musically induced highs" may be caused by a shot of endorphins released on musical command into the bloodstream. Dr. Ralph Spintge (1983), one of the speakers at this symposium, reported that he and his medical associates in West Germany have observed the effects of anxiety-reducing music, self-selected by dental surgery patients for the purpose of inducing anlagesia. The medicinal effect was the reduction in blood levels of the stress hormone ACTH (adrenocorticopichormone), and the raising of the endogenous opiod, beta-endorphin. Some kinds of music can produce in the brain the same "feel-good" chemicals that may occur from running (runner's high) or meditation (alpha state-centered). As such, they can reduce the intensity of the pain a person may be experiencing. Crow (1984) reported that music and other stimuli can produce another neurochemical, phenylethylamine, in the human system. Klein and Liebowitz (1984) have labelled PEA the chemical of love because it produces the euphoric "falling in love" type of feeling.

Wood (1984) reported in the *University of California, Berkeley Wellness Letter:*

> I well remember a few years ago playing in a 'Ludwig Fest' in Denver. On that program we performed all nine of the Beethoven symphonies in one day. It was such an exhausting project that all I could think of before was 'Will I get through it?' At the end of the 'Sixth Symphony' I was ready to fold up. Then, the next one, the marvelous 'Seventh' was conducted by William Smith of the Philadelphia Orchestra. Under Smith, the Seventh Symphony came to life and, at the end of it, I felt much better. I got through the 'Eighth' in good shape, and, then, Smith conducted the 'Ninth.' I was so excited and inspired by that, even though we had played for hours and hours, I could have gladly

played it again right then. But what surprised me most was what I felt the day after and the week after. I have never before or since experienced the 'lift' I felt. I was almost in another world.

Another area of interest is the connection between visualization, imagery, or mind and bodily functions. Ever since Hans Seyle began his studies dealing with the phenomena of "stress," interest has mushroomed in techniques and procedures to reduce stress levels as a source of preventive medicine. More recently, the fief of psychoneuroimmunology has been accepted as a reputable field of scientific study. Penfield (   ) and other neurosurgeons have conducted studies of the temporal lobes that indicate a possible correlation between music and imagery or visualization. Their research has shown that removal of portions of the right temporal lobe reduce or toally destroy visualization ability. Since the first split brain studies of the early 1960s, research in hemispheric specialization has indicated that most people, with the exception of trained musicians, process music largely through the right temporal lobe. Therefore, if studies such as those conducted by Nicholas Hall of George Washington University, Washington, D.C., show that visualization or imagery can serve as a source for developing positive immune responses, then it is possible that music may be an adjunct to facilitate visualization therapy. Hall (1984) reports:

> . . . During the practice to positive imagery--that is, of imagining one's immune system attacking one's tumor--there was a synchronous rise both in the number of lymphocytes circulating in the peripheral blood and in blood serum levels of the thymic hormone thymosin alpha. The increased values suffered a decline during periods when the patient did not practice positive imagery.

Hammer (1984), Yates (1980), and Adler (1981) report other studies in the area of visualization. Current subliminal tapes and guided imagery tapes utilize the positive reinforcing benefits of music to facilitate and even generate imagery that can, in turn, strengthen natural immune responses.

Rider (1985) et al. of Eastern Montana College measured the effects of music, progressive muscle relaxation, and guided imagery on the adrenal corticosteroids, or "stress hormones." Their research was based on the fact that the adrenal cortex produces/releases large amounts of corticosterone (steroids) during periods of stress. The effects of continued exposure of the large amounts of corticosteroids upon the immune system have been shown to be quite detrimental. Therefore, their study showed that because music, imagery, and relaxation (PMR) can affect stress hormones, there is an indirect link that can be drawn to immune response levels through the therapeutic uses of music, imagery, and relaxation. A second aspect of their study was to test whether or not stress (which is related to disease) can be caused by a state of desynchronization of the himan circadian oscillators. Such oscillators include body temperature, electrolytes, corticosteroids, and neurotransmitters, each of which demonstrates a daily periodic rhythm. The hypothalmic system of the brain controls the response level to stress and is the seat of circadian patterning. Rider et al. report the implication of their study is:

> . . . that a technique exists using music listening to alter body chemistry in positive directions. Such chronic diseases as the autoimmune syndromes and cancer, as well as the more acute viral infections, need to be studied to determine their responsivity to such techniques. The stress-reducing properties of music/PMR/GI have more obvious implications for use in mental health and educational settings. Further research should investigate the complete role of music in facilitating imagery and relaxation and should attempt to determine which of the three components is most important to general health.

The scope of this topic necessitates a severe limiting in the sharing of further studies that illustrate a direct or possible correlation between music and health. This is an expanding area of interest for many participants at this symposium. Given proper research and clinical environment, and private and professional support for further studies, within a few years, many questions raised during this symposium will have answers, and new questions will be generated.

Music has many functions at this time in history. We can utilize it in our culture as a source of individual and group health, as long as we become aware of both the positive and negative effects of sound. Music can be a source of ineffable communication, a vehicle for experiential and vicarious catharsis, and an aid for either an individual or group environment for renewing sound. Music can also aid in the following biological functions: digestion, facilitation of relaxation and visualization, energizing of both psychic and physical being, and facilitation of emotional homeostatis. Music can complement and enhance physical, chemical, and mental treatment modalities. It can serve as a bridge between: the known and the unknown, the conscious and the unconscious, the physical and the metaphysical, the singular and

83

the universal, the temporal and the spiritual, and the scientific and the artistic.

In the context of this paper and within the scope of this symposium, it is proposed that music can be, ought to be, and, hopefully, one day will be an integral part of the healing arts dedicated to wholeness for all mankind.

REFERENCES

Ader, R. (1981). *Psychoneuroimmunology.* New York: Academic Press.

Bailey, L. M. (1983). The effects of live music versus tape-recorded music on hospitalized cancer patients. *Music Therapy, 3,* 17-28.

Bonny, H. L. (1983). Music listening for intensive coronary care units: A pilot project. *Music Therapy, 3,* 4-16.

Brody, R. (1984, April). Music medicine. *Omni, 24,* 110.

Buckingham, C. (1983, September). Music mellows radiation therapy. *The Messenger, 12,* 3.

Chetta, H. D. (1981). The effect of music and desensitization on preoperative anxiety in children. *Journal of Music Therapy, 18,* 74-87.

Clark, M., McCorkle, R., & Williams, S. (1981). Music therapy-assisted labor and delivery. *Journal of Music Therapy, 18,* 88-100.

Crow, P. (1984, May 21), Waking up the right lobe. *Vital Speeches of the Day,* pp. 600-601.

Diamond, J. (1981). *The life energy in music: Notes on music and sound* (2 vols.). Valley Cottage, New York: Archaeus Press.

Gewirtz, M. H. (1978). Research on the impact of the healing arts. In Howard Klein (Ed.) *The healing role of the arts.* New York: The Rockefeller Foundation.

Goldstein, A. (1985, Jan. 21/Feb. 11). Music/endorphin link. *Brain/Mind Bulletin, 2,* 1.

Hanser, S. L., & O'Connell, A. (1983). The effect of music on relaxation of expectant mothers during labor. *Journal of Music Therapy, 20,* 50-58.

Hall, N. R. (1984). A workshop on positive emotions. *Advances, 1,* 5-6.

Halpern, S., & Savary, L. (1985). *Sound health.* New York: Harper & Row.

Hammer, Signe. (1984, April). The mind as healer. *Science Digest,* 47-49;100.

Harvey, A. (1985). Understanding your brain's response to music. *International Brain Dominance Review, 2:1*, 32-39.

Hoy, R. (1972, November). Recordings for recovery: A service to humanity. *Music Journal, 42*, 13-14.

Kabat-Zinn, J. (n.d.). *The stress reduction and relaxation program.* Unpublished manuscript, University of Massachusetts Medical Center, Worcester, Massachusetts.

Kuemmel, W. (1977). *Musik und medizin.* Freiburg/Muenchen: Karl Alber.

Livingood, A., Kiser, K., & Paige, N. (1984). *A study of families to determine the effect of sedate music on their state anxiety level while they await the outcome of surgery.* Unpublished research project, Eastern Kentucky University, Richmond, Kentucky.

Livingston, J. C. (1979 November/December). Music for the Childbearing family. *Journal of Obstetric and Gynecological Nursing, 17*, 363-367.

MacClelland, D. C. (1979). Music in the operating room. *AORN Journal, 29*, 252-260.

Malesky, G. (1983, October). Music that strikes a healing chord. *Prevention, 35:10*, pp. 57-63.

Marley, L. (1984). The use of music with hospitalized infants and toddlers: A descriptive study. *Journal of Music Therapy, 21*, 126-132.

Muzak. (n.d.a). *Music in the preoperative holding area.* Unpublished music research note no. 51, Creighton University/St. Joseph's Hospital, Yonkers, New York.

Muzak. (n.d.b). *Muzak joins the surgical team at union hospital.* Unpublished file no. 1732, Union Hospital, Bronx, New York.

Muzak. (n.d.c). Programmed muzak for the coronary patient. In *Environs*, reprinted by permission of publisher, New York: Muzak, A Division of Teleprompter Corporation.

Muzak. (1982). *Proof! Muzak produces measurable results.* Unpublished Summary Report, Muzak, A Division of Telepromter Corporation.

Penfield, W. (1975). *The mystery of the mind: A critical study of consciousness and the human brain*. Princeton, New Jersey: Princeton University Press.

Pratt, R. R. (1985). The historical relationship between music and medicine. In R. R. Pratt (Ed.), *The Third International Symposium on Music in Medicine, Education, and Therapy for the Handicapped* (pp. 237-269). Lanham, Maryland: University Press of America.

Rosenbaum, R. (1984, June). The chemistry of love. *Esquire*, pp. 100-111.

Rider, M., Floyd, J., & Kirkpatrick, J. (1985). The effect of music, imagery, and relaxation on adrenal corticosteroids and the reentrainment of circadian rhythms. *Journal of Music Therapy*, *22*, 46-58.

Klein, H. (Ed.). (1978). *The healing role of the arts*. New York: The Rockefeller Foundation.

Salk, L. (1981). Mother's beat as an imprinting stimulus. In R. O. Benezon (Ed.), *Music Therapy Manual* (pp. 22-24). Springfield, Illinois: Charles C. Thomas.

Schullian, D., & Schoen, M. (Eds.). (1948). *Music and medicine*. New York: Henry Schuman.

Shanahy, E. (1984). Music for a healthy heart. *Keyboard Classics*, *6*, 4-5.

Spintge, R. & Droh, R. (Eds.). (1985). *Music in Medicine Proceedings II. International Symposium "Music in Medicine," Ludenscheid 1984*, Schattauer: Stuttgart: Roche.

Taylor, D. (1981). Music in general hospital treatment from 1900-1950. *Journal of Music Therapy, 18*, 62-73.

Verny, T., & Kelly, J. (1982). *The secret life of the unborn child*. New York: Dell Publishing Co.

Wood, A. (1985). Stokowski encore. *University of California/Berkeley Wellness Letter, 1:8*, pp. 6-7.

Yates, J. (1980, April). Thoughts that heal. *Prevention, 32:4*, pp. 58-64.

EFFECTS OF ANXIOLYTIC MUSIC ON PLASMA LEVELS OF STRESS HORMONES IN DIFFERENT MEDICAL SPECIALITIES

by

RALPH SPINTGE and ROLAND DROH

The Pyschophysical State of the Patient

Patients endure a certain amount of psychic and physical distress whenever they are either waiting for medical treatment or experiencing the treatment itself. This holds true both in clinical situations and with ambulatory patients treated in private practice. The distress, independent of the basic disease, always brings on significant irritation to the whole body.

Why does a patient visit a doctor? The main complaints are anxiety and pain. Some of the most important pathophysiological implications of anxiety and pain are:

1. Arrhythmias, angina pectoris, hypertension, hyperventilation, and even asthma, which occur in the cardiopulmonary system
2. A lowered threshold of pain tolerance and a general hyperesthesis
3. Increased muscle tension and excitement
4. The rising of plasma levels of catecholamines, steroids, and endogenous opiods
5. Imparied subjective feeling of the patient that in turn creates inadequate defense reactions and reduces compliance
6. An increased demand for anxiolytic and analgesic drugs

Physicians must try to influence the psychophysical situation of the patient in order to avoid these undesirable reactions. It has become clear that pharmaceutical and psychological means alone are not sufficient nor can they be used in many cases. One explanation for this is that many fears cannot be treated with rational arguments.

There is usually no time for individual and sensitive conversation in the daily routine between doctor and patient, especially when anesthesiology and surgery are involved. Many patients are so overwhelmed by their fears that they are unable to gain any emotional profit from their talks with the physician. This is one reason for the widely used patient information booklets, which the patient has to read and sign.

The psychophysical situation of the patient can be described by the term "regression." And this regression needs some kind of a nonverbal communication that at least can establish an emotional connection with the patient. Psychotherapists have told us that music can accomplish this goal.

In addition to the anxiety-creating stimuli, the patient also suffers from a certain lack of stimulation from his normal environment. He is separated from his family, his friends, his company, etc. In order to live in psychological and physiological harmony, a person needs a certain level of stimulation that comes from a normal life situation. Music that is familiar to the patient can, in this sense, be a bridge to the normal life situation. Young patients, for example, use disco music to escape to the environment they obviously like most.

For the last eight years our research team has conducted several clinically controlled and randomized studies in different medical specialties like anesthesiology, surgery, orthopedics, dentistry, and obstetrics.

Method

The procedure for using anxiolytic music in all these different specialties is quite similar. The following is a description of the procedure as it is used in anesthesiology and surgery.

On the day before the operation, the patient receives a preoperative questionnaire asking not only about his medical anamnesis but also his musical preferences.

Nearly 50,000 patients examined during the years 1977-1985 were given five categories of music from which to choose. The following table shows their selections:

TABLE 1

FREQUENCY OF CHOICE PERCENTAGES
AMONG 50,000 PATIENTS

Music Category	Frequency of Choice %
Popular Music ("James Last happy sound")	44%
Soft Popular Music	6%
Classics (mainly from the Romantic Period)	15%
Military Music	10%
Actual Pop Hits	25%
% of Patients Satisfied with This Selection	95%

On the morning of the operation the patient is wheeled into the preoperation waiting area and given earphones to listen to the music he has selected. In cases where general anesthesia is administered, the earphones are worn until the patient is asleep. Where local anesthesia is given, the patient listens to music throughout the entire operation. As part of the postoperative procedure, the patient receives another questionnaire about his subjective feelings concerning the operation, anesthesia, postoperative complaints and, of course, the music.

Results

Studies conducted since 1982 indicate that patients listening to music of their choice during certain medical procedures experience better psychophysical effects than those who do not have the musical stimuli.[1] Figures 1 - 8 show some physiological and endocrinological effects of anxiolytic music during dental treatment, surgery in epidural anesthesia, and during labor. These results are replicated in all our studies and show a statistically significant reduction (p<.01) of stress response in the cardiovascular and endocrinological systems.

Definition and Precondition of Anxiolytic Music

The term "anxiolytic music", as used in all these studies, is a pragmatic and empirical one. Music is "anxiolytic" if it has the desired psychological and physiological effects mentioned above. The following preconditions, however, must be fulfilled:

1. Musical works should be selected according to duration, instrumentation, dynamics, and interpretation. It is important that there be no extremes in rhythm, melody, or dynamics; more lower than higher frequencies; a frequency range from 100 - 10,000 Hz; and that instrumental (preferably strings) rather than vocal music be chosen
2. Patients should make their own musical selections
3. The effects of individual pieces and combinations of pieces should be tested in ongoing clinical settings
4. Recordings should be of high quality, yet technically simple and reliable

(It is most important that the patient, not the doctor or nurse, choose the music. Pieces chosen by the patient should then be screened for a final selection of familiar melodies and simple rhythmic structures. Instrumental music is to be preferred since vocal lyrics induce arousal reactions that are counterproductive to the desired state of relaxation. The only exception to this last rule is in the case of pop music. The reason for this exception is that in most cases no one understands what the pop artist is singing anyway.) Among the classics, violin, flute, and piano music is more suitable than works featuring instruments such as the trumpet,

---

[1]Ralph Spintge, "Psychologische und psychotherapeutische Methoden zur Verminderung praeoperativer Angst," M.D. dissertation, University of Bonn Faculty of Medicine, 1982; Roland Droh and Ralph Spintge, eds., *Angst, Schmerz und Musik in der Anaesthesie* (Grenzach: Editiones Roche, 1983); Ralph Spintge and Roland Droh, eds., *Music in Medicine: 2. International Symposion Sportkrankenhaus Hellersen Luedenscheid/Deutschland* (Grenzach: Editiones Roche, 1985).

Effect of Anxiolytic Music
on Pulse Rate in Dental Procedure

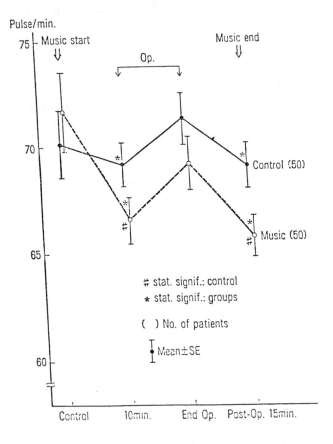

Figure 1

**Effect of Anxiolytic Music on Pulse Rate
in Dental Procedure**

Control group and music group, 50 patients each. Statistically significant differences between control group and music group after 10 minutes from the start of the music (during dental treatment) and 15 minutes after the end of the dental treatment. T. Oyama, K. Hatano, Y. Sato, M. Kudo, Ralph Spintge, and Roland Droh, "Endocrine Effect of Anxiolytic Music in Dental Patients," in *Angst, Schmerz und Musik*, eds. Roland Droh and Ralph Spintge (Grenzach: Editiones Roche, 1983), pp. 143-46.

92

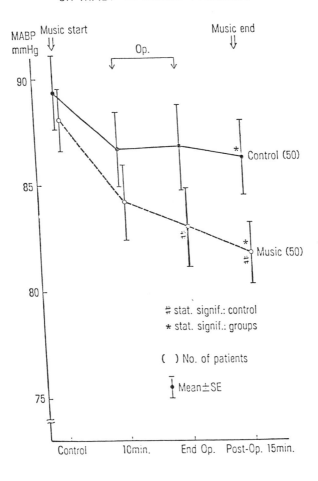

Figure 2

Effect of Anxiolytic Music on Mean Arterial Blood
Pressure MABP in Dental Procedure
(same study as in Figure 1)

Effect of Anxiolytic Music
on Plasma ACTH Levels in Dental Procedure

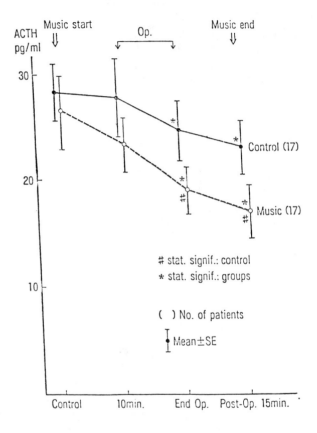

Figure 3

Effect of Anxiolytic Music on Plasma Adrenocorticotrophic
Hormone ACTH Levels in Dental Procedure
(same study as in Figure 1)

94

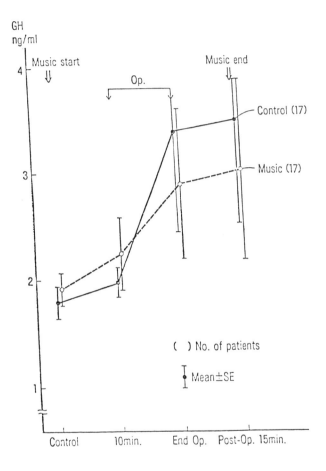

Effect of Anxiolytic Music
on Plasma GH Levels in Dental Procedure

Figure 4

Effect of Anxiolytic Music on Plasma Growth Hormone
Levels GH in Dental Procedure
(same study as in Figure 1)

Effect of Anxiolytic Music
on Plasma PRL Levels in Dental Procedure

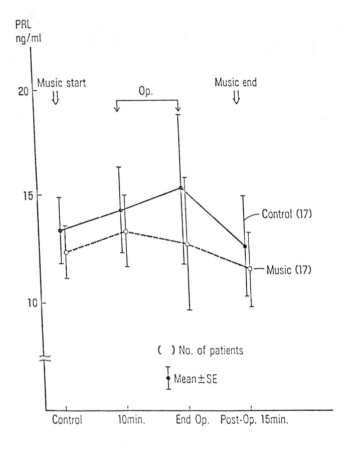

Figure 5

Effect of Anxiolytic Music on Plasma Prolactin
Levels PRL in Dental Procedure
(same study as in Figure 1)

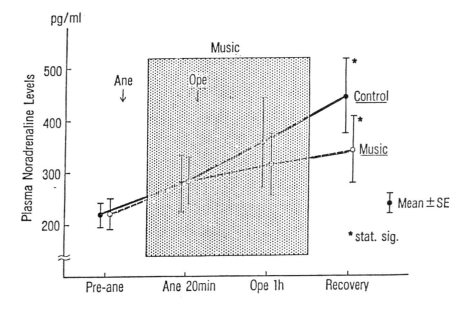

Figure 6

Effect of Music on Plasma Levels of Noradrenaline in
Surgical Patients with Epidural Anaesthesia

Control group and music group 15 patients each. Statistically
significant differences after 1 hour of operation and during postoperative recovery period. F. Tanioka, T. Takazawa, S. Kamata, M.
Kudo, A. Matsuki, T. Oyama: "Hormonal Effect of Anxiolytic Music
in Patients During Surgical Operations Under Epidural Anaesthesia"
in *Music in Medicine*, eds. Ralph Spintge and Roland Droh
(Grenzach: Editiones Roches, 1985), pp. 285-290.

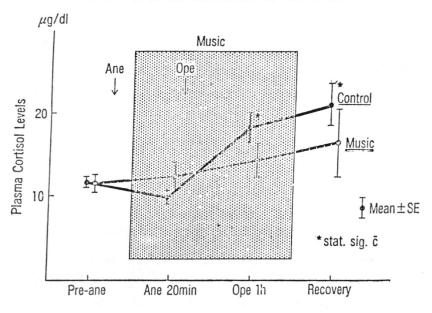

Figure 7

Effect of Music on Plasma Levels of Cortisol
(same study as in Figure 6)

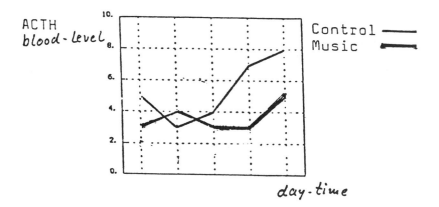

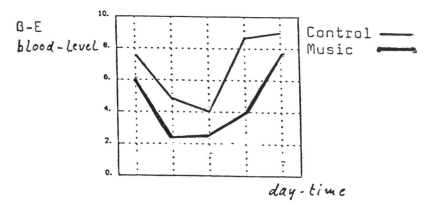

Figure 8

Effect of Music on Plasma ACTH-Levels and Plasma B-Endorphine -
Levels During Labor Over the Course of a 24 Hour Day

Control group and music group 100 women each. Statistically
significant differences (p< 0.002) between control group and music
group demonstrate a remarkable stress reducing effect of music. B.
Halpaap, R. Spintge, R. Droh, W. Kummert, W. Koegel, "Anxiolytic
Music in Obstetrics," in *Music in Medicine*, eds. Ralph Spintge and
Roland Droh (Grenzach: Editiones Roche, 1985), pp. 145-154. If
military music is chosen, however, trumpets and drums contribute
to the desired effect, creating some kind of an inner discipline.

Conclusion

To date, anxiolytic music has been tried in many different medical procedures such as anesthesia, surgery, dentistry, obstetrics, psychotherapy, intensive care medicine, therapy with drug addicts, and pain therapy.

Our data show that no undesirable side effects occur if music is used properly. On the contrary, the data suggest that there may be no medical procedure where music cannot be used for the benefit of the patient.

REFERENCES

Droh, Roland, and Spintge, Ralph, eds. *Angst, Schmerz und Musik in der Anaesthesie.* Grenzach: Editiones Roche, 1983.

Spintge, Ralph. "Psychologische und psychotherapeutische Methoden zur Verminderung praeoperativer Angst." M.D. dissertation, University of Bonn Faculty of Medicine, 1982.

Spintge, Ralph, and Droh, Roland, eds. *Music in Medicine:* 2. International Symposion Sport krankenhaus Hellersen Luedenscheid/Deutschland. Grenzach: Editiones Roche, 1985.

MUSICAL OPTIONS FOR UPPER-LIMB AMPUTEES

by

JOAN E. EDELSTEIN

Imagination and ingenuity can initiate individuals with upper-limb amputation into the pleasure of musical participation. Musicianship not only fosters self-expression and self-confidence, but it also can improve coordination and respiratory function. Some amputees participate in a musical activity by means of a prosthesis, while others do not wear such a device when playing selected instruments. In other instances, simple adaptations can unlock the treasure of instrumental music. With emphasis on a musical theme, the following information is arranged by instrumental groups in order to demonstrate prospects for upper-limb amputees in every kind of orchestral and band ensemble.

Brass Instruments

The slide trombone is particularly suited to unilateral amputees at any level as well as to bilateral below-elbow (BE) amputees who wear prostheses. The unilateral amputee grasps the slide with the intact hand and supports the instrument with the prosthetic hook or artificial hand. In the case of amputation on the right side, the trombonist switches hands, supporting with the right prosthesis and sliding with the left limb. Advanced BE players, who must support and slide with a prosthesis, can produce slide vibrato by delicate elbow motion. Amputees may use a post or counterbalances to help support the weight of the trombone. Difficulty in assembling the instrument can be reduced by asking a friend to assist or by removing the prostheses in order to use the broader, more resilient surfaces of the bare amputation limbs, then redonning the prostheses to play.

A bugle is another valveless instrument well suited to amputees. It can be supported and played by any unilateral amputee or a bilateral BE amputee with or without prostheses, or a bilateral above-elbow (AE) amputee wearing at least one prosthesis. The bugle can be held on either side, thus opening up the fun of marching in fife-drum-bugle corps to limb-deficient children or adults.

Valved instruments are also accessible to the amputee. The valved trombone lends itself to switch-hand playing in the case of the right BE or AE amputee, who would support the trombone with the right prosthesis and press the valves with the left hand. The trumpet and cornet are more popular instruments that can be played with either hand. In order to play these instruments, the prosthesis is hooked into the top ring. There are several ways to keep the hook from scratching the brass finish: (1) the appropriate part of the trumpet may be covered with masking tape; or (2) the hook itself may be covered with rubber tubing or Plastisol coating.

Without a prosthesis, the BE trumpeter supports the instrument on the amputated limb, and the AE amputee can use a custom-made stand or adapted neck strap. One bilateral BE musician sits in such a way that he can prop the bell on his thigh and depress the valves with either or both amputation limbs. He uses both limbs for valves one and three, and either limb for any one or two adjacent valves. In this manner, he can play fast enough to produce sixteenth notes. The individual who has at least three functional digits on either hand can play in the normal manner.

Although the French horn player normally depresses the valves with the left hand and stops the bell with the right, left side amputees can do the reverse. Right BE amputees use the bare amputation limb in the bell, a technique used by several professional hornists who are also right side amputees. If the musician prefers to wear a prosthesis, a transposing mute can be helpful. The baritone, alto horn, and mellophone are traditionally right-handed instruments that can be played in reverse by unilateral right BE and AE amputees. Larger brass instruments, such as the tuba and Sousaphone, are suitable for unilateral left amputees. The lightweight fiberglass tuba or the regular Sousaphone are easier to carry than the conventional tuba. The instruments can also be supported on the lap on commercially available chair stands.

Percussion

Percussion offers many opportunities for vigorous displays of musicianship. Preschoolers, grasping a terminal device, join their peers in shaking tone bells, tambourines, maracas, and similar instruments. Without a prosthesis, the BE amputee holds the instrument in the antecubital fossa and the AE amputee uses the axilla. More sophisticated percussionists use the terminal device of the prosthesis to hold strikers or mallets for the triangle, xylophone, vibraphone, marimba, glockenspiel, and bell lyre.

Larger instruments are supported on floor stands while a table or neck strap suffices for the lighter ones. The sustaining pedal of the vibraphone makes it especially rewarding for unilateral or bilateral BE and AE amputees. One jazz and rock drummer who wears bilateral shoulder disarticulation prostheses creates complex rhythms by means of trunk and scapular motion. His special prostheses have rigid shoulder joints, elbow units locked at ninety degrees, and locked turntables. His drum sticks are notched to fit the hook tines, and wide rubber tubing holds the sticks in place. In this manner, he is able to perform professionally on the trap set, snare and bass drums, tympani, gongs, chimes, and the rest of the battery. The pedal-operated bass drum poses no problem for the seated amputee. When marching in a parade, the drummer can have an excellent experience by holding the sticks in the terminal device(s). For band participation, harness adaptations may be necessary to enable amputee musicians to keep in step. Crash cymbals are an obvious favorite of prosthesis wearers.

The piano, organ, harpsichord, and similar keyboard instruments are well within the reach of individuals with upper-limb disorders. The virtuosity of Paul Wittgenstein, the concert artist who sustained traumatic right amputation during World War I, serves as inspiration to pianists. Soon after his injury, he discovered works for the left hand by Haydn, and Godowsky's arrangements for left hand of nineteen Chopin etudes. He arranged many compositions himself and later commissioned Ravel, Prokofiev, Strauss, Hindemith, and Britten to compose literature that is still programmed in today's concert halls. There is also piano music for one hand that is on an elementary level, and resourceful music teachers can arrange many selections that will provide satisfaction for the one-handed artist.

Another keyboard technique, this time for the right BE amputee, involves the use of the bare amputation limb to strike one key while the thumb of the intact hand adds a second note to the treble chord, and the fingers of the left hand play the bass line. This technique affords greater sensory feedback and freedom of movement through direct contact with the keys, although G-sharp poses some difficulties. Clearly, pieces written in the keys of C, G, and F major are the easiest because they use the fewest black keys. Several children with bilateral congenital deficiencies play by holding rubber-tipped pencils or dowels in the axillae.

Unilateral or bilateral amputees can wear a piano terminal device that consists of aluminum tubing, seven inches long and curved to span an octave when the hook is opened fully. The metal is covered with rubber or resilient plastic to protect the keys. An alternate prosthetic approach involves simply covering the middle finger of the prosthetic hand with a bookkeeper's rubber finger cot to extend the finger enough so that the pianist can strike the keys accurately. The sustaining pedal of the piano allows even the beginner to produce full-sounding music even if only single notes are played.

The chord organ and electric piano are economical options. The left amputee will have little difficulty because the buttons are usually on the left side, allowing the right hand to play the keyboard. The right amputee plays by crossing hands. The compactness of electronic keyboards makes these instruments easy to play when placed across a wheelchair lapboard or on a bed table. The great variety of sonic effects now available should satisfy musicians of every kind.

The piano accordion can be played in a reverse manner, or, as with the piano, the keyboard can be struck with a rubber-tipped hook, middle finger of the prosthetic hand, or the bare BE amputation limb. Three digits are normally needed to play the chord buttons.

The autoharp can be strummed with either hand while the bare amputation limb depresses the chord bar or holds the pick secured in a snug band around the limb or in a prosthetic terminal device. The instrument can be supported on the lap or a table. The harmonica is another instrument available to the amputee, who can purchase a neck holder in any instrument store.

Stringed Instruments

Performance on the violin and viola is attainable if the player's commitment to diligent practice is complemented by careful instrument selection and simple adaptations. The right amputee can finger the strings in the usual manner, while the unilateral left amputee can manage if the strings, and sometimes the bridge, are reversed. Bowing is accomplished by the partial hand amputee who has a bow-holding opposition post. Individuals with BE amputation can wear a prosthetic hand equipped with a special bow holder that permits the bow to swivel without sliding from the prosthesis. The instrument is supported with the aid of a prosthetic harness, altered to make it rather snug. The cello is even more accessible because it is easier to support on the floor and the bow strokes are broader. The same bow holder is suitable.

The most popular stringed instrument is the electric or acoustic guitar. The right BE amputee performs in the customary manner, holding the pick in the terminal device or in a snug bracelet fitted on the bare amputation limb. The AE guitarist must substitute shoulder motion for elbow and forearm motion in order to move the pick. Left amputees simply reverse the strings and bridge or play cross handed. Commercial guitars for the left hand are another possibility. Comparable techniques can be tried by aspiring string bassists, particularly for performance of popular pieces that use a pizzicato technique. Electric guitars generally have the tuning pegs on one side; for the left-hand model, the pegs are moved to the opposite side. Other stringed instruments such as the banjo, ukelele, mandolin, Hawaiian guitar, and dulcimer can also be played in reverse manner. Some dulcimer players hold the strings with the bare amputation limb, one finger, or a rubber-tipped dowel while strumming with the intact hand. The bilateral amputee can hold a plectrum in the prosthesis or strapped to the BE limb.

Woodwinds

Although the least suitable for the individual with major amputation, the flute, piccolo, oboe, English horn, clarinet, and saxophone can be played by partial hand amputees if the loss is limited to the right thumb, which ordinarily is used to help support the instrument and not for the keys. A hand opposition post plus a neck strap or the knees can help support the instrument. One BE professional square dance caller holds a penny flute in his antecubital fossa and is able to play with ease.

Coda

Alternatives to instrumental performance are an invitation to the prospective musician. A splendid example was set by Robert Schumann, who continued in music in spite of an injury in the third and fourth fingers of his right hand caused by a mechanical finger strengthener he had invented. Schumann's genius as a composer has enriched the musical world immeasurably. On a contemporary note, many phases of audioengineering are feasible for some upper limb amputees. Of course, manual dexterity is not a prerequisite for singing, and many amputees find and give great pleasure vocalizing in popular and classical ensembles and as professional and amateur soloists.

The harmonious interaction of qualified music instructors and clinical personnel can bring the joy of musical participation to anyone who is interested, regardless of the number or character of the musician's limbs.

REFERENCES

Ballantyne, J. "Schumann's Hand Injury." *British Medical Journal* 1 (1978):1142-

Elliott, B. *Guide to the Selection of Musical Instruments with Respect to Physical Ability and Disability.* Philadelphia, Pennsylvania: Moss Rehabilitation Hospital, 1982.

Erickson, L. "Keyboard Fun for Children with Osteogenesis Imperfecta and Other Physical Limitations." *Inter-Clinic Information Bulletin* 12 (January 1973):9-16.

_____. "Never Say 'You Can't Do That' to an Amputee!" *Inter-Clinic Information Bulletin* 13 (July 1974):13-14.

_____. "Piano Playing as a Hobby for Children with Problem Hands." *Inter-Clinic Information Bulletin* 11 (March 1972):6-17.

Henson, R. A., and Ulrich, H. "Schumann's Hand Injury." *British Medical Journal* 1 (1978):900-903.

Kral, C. "Musical Instruments for Upper-Limb Amputees." *Inter-Clinic Information Bulletin* 12 (December 1972):13-26.

Mailhot, A. "Musical Instruments for Upper-Limb Amputees." *Inter-Clinic Information Bulletin* 13 (July 1974):9-15.

Musical Instruments for the Limb-Deficient Child. A motion picture. Los Angeles, California: University of California at Los Angeles, 1977.

Riccardi, J., and Vella, A. *Elementary Piano for One Hand.* Boston, Massachussetts: Boston Music Company, n.d.

THE PHYSICAL INJURY (OVERUSE) DUE TO MUSIC MAKING

by

HUNTER J. H. FRY

Introduction

It is now generally recognized that music making is able to cause physical damage in the player.[1] This involves the motor units of the upper limb, mouth, palate, upper respiratory tract, and spine. This condition is now increasingly known as "overuse injury": overuse, because it appears to be produced by long, intensive, and excessive muscular activity; and injury, because the more serious examples show evidence of tissue damage, and loss of function.

Many handicapped people now turn to music to enhance their quality of life. At the opening ceremony of this fourth MEH conference, Carol Gardiner showed what could be done with her choir of wheelchair patients. The Honorary President of this association, Itzhak Perlman, has taken his rightful place among the great musicians of the twentieth century, notwithstanding his disablement.

It clearly behooves us to protect the handicapped person against the hazards of music making as they are known, for a handicapped person does not need yet another handicap. Education and understanding the nature of the overuse process and its prevention are the means by which the handicapped person can be so protected.

Definition

Overuse injury can be defined as a painful condition of the upper limb, produced by intensive or prolonged use of the limb and use that is excessive for the individuals affected. This definition can be extended to the muscle units used in embouchure, the soft palate dividing the roof of the mouth from the floor of the nose,

---

[1]Hunter J. H. Fry, "Occupational Maladies of Musicians: Their Cause and Prevention," *International Journal of Music Education* 2 (November 1984):63-66; idem, "Physical Signs in the Hand and Wrist Seen in the Overuse Injury Syndrome of the Upper Limb," *Australian and New Zealand Journal of Surgery,* in press; idem, "Overuse Injury Syndrome in the Upper Limb in Musicians," *Medical Journal of Australia* 144, no. 4 (1986):182-85.

the muscles of the throat, and the muscles of the spine. The same condition is seen in other hand-use intense activities. The fast electronic keyboards, such as word processors and video display units and computor terminals, produce a great many such injuries. The condition may also be contracted by the assembly line worker in industry, the writer, and the potter.[2] Parallel studies of the condition in these other occupations give insights into the musician's problem that would not otherwise be possible.

The writer's present study began about two years ago when problems of musician patients could not be reconciled with commonly accepted explanations of their symptoms. There are four such notions: Tendinitis (Tenosynovitis), a collection of unrelated disorders, "it's all in the mind," and bad teaching and "misuse."

Tendinitis (Tenosynovitis)

Tendinitis means inflammation of tendons or tendon sheaths. There are also other words meaning nearly the same thing. While most people would agree that the trouble is in the motor units, these terms specify that the injury or process is in the tendon, which is the toughest part of the muscle fiber and does not itself contract.

Tendinitis and tenosynovitis do exist in both the hand and the foot and constitute a *specific condition that is easily verified*. It is exemplified in the hand by trigger finger, trigger thumb, and deQuervain's disease, which affects the tendon sheath of some of the thumb tendons on that side of the wrist. Tenosynovitis can occur in rheumatoid disease and may be responsible for actual rupture of the tendons on the back of the wrist. These forms of true tenosynovitis are treated by surgical intervention wherein a portion of the tendon sheath is removed so that the tendon can glide freely; this usually cures the trouble. In the case of rheumatoid disease, the mass of tissue is removed to protect the tendons from further attack. When the tendon and tendon sheaths are exposed at operation, any abnormality is readily *apparent on naked eye examination* and is *highly photogenic*. When tissue is removed (and this is generally the case) at operation, it can be sent to the pathology laboratory where it is processed, stained, and examined under a microscope, *clearly showing the underlying condition*.

---

[2]Idem, "Overuse Injury in Potters," *Pottery in Australia* 24, no. 3 (September 1985):48-50.

Even at this point, the naked eye appearance and the microscopic anatomy of the condition in the hand and wrist have not been displayed in overuse injury. Such evidence is a basic requirement before the existence of the condition in tendons can be accepted. On these grounds alone, it is unproven. Because overuse injury in musicians has been so refractory to treatment, and because the label for the disorder has been accepted, the patient resorts to surgery out of desperation. As a result, many musicians, and still more patients in other occupations with the same condition, have been subjected to operations without positive findings. This effectively disproves this commonly accepted diagnosis and renders it meaningless. A misleading diagnosis is worse than no diagnosis at all, for treatment must become a matter of "hit and miss," and notions of prevention become problematical. Along with this notion of tendinitis (tenosynovitis) comes the implicit assumption that this is an *inflammatory condition,* and this, too, has *never been proven.*

A Collection of Unrelated Disorders

Some people still hold to the view that overuse injury is really a collection of unrelated disorders that are themselves not common but, together, explain what is happening.[3] These conditions include carpal tunnel syndrome; ulna nerve neuropathy; other nerve entrapment syndromes, including thoracic outlet syndrome, reflex sympathetic dystrophy, and osteoarthritis at the base of the thumb. With the exception of thoracic outlet syndrome, these conditions are all relatively uncommon, well understood, and, for the most part, treated surgically. Thoracic outlet syndrome is highly contentious and difficult to prove one way or the other. Patients with overuse injury present symptoms and signs that are impossible to reconcile with tolerably well understood, specific conditions.

"It's All in the Mind"

It is somewhat unfortunate that many musicians and individuals from other occupations who experience pain in the upper limbs are told that there is nothing wrong with them and that it is really something that is being imagined and is not real. Advice of this kind is very stressful and can only act in a negative way. Since the condition is now well known and is usually

---

[3]C. D. Browne, B. M. Nolan, and D. K. Faithfull, "Occupational Repetition Strain Injuries: Guidelines for Diagnosis and Management," *Medical Journal of Australia* 140 (March 1984):329-32.

accompanied by reproducible physical signs, it is important to retain balance about any psychological element that is present. Kimber has claimed that musicians have converted fear of failure and uncoordination into pain.[4] He also claimed that the viola section of a particular orchestra (which he would not name) took turns off playing, a process which he said the players worked out among themselves. Neither this nor his conversion disorder theory can be supported, for he was not able to quote any basis for his claims nor is such a basis to be found anywhere in the literature. One criterion for diagnosis of conversion disorder is that there is no adequate physical explanation for the conversion.[5] The other criterion is the presence of a demonstrable psychological dynamic responsible for the conversion mechanism. Since that is not the case in overuse injury (also called a repetition strain injury), the proposition immediately falls down. The presentation of these musician patients is quite incompatible with the psychiatric salad imaginatively described by Kimber, himself an amateur pianist.

Indeed, Hochberg, Leffert, and Newmark from Massachussetts General Hospital report less than 1% incidence of psychiatric illness in their musician patients.[6] Lederman from the Cleveland Clinic does not report any and, in the writer's series, would certainly be below 5%.[7]

Bad Teaching and "Misuse"

These allegations, which blame either the teacher for bad teaching or the student for "misuse," are unfortunate for several reasons. While it is perhaps comforting to apportion blame to clearly identifiable people or objects, these allegations have the

---

[4]W. Kimber, "R.S.I. and Musicians," *Victoria Ministry of the Arts Seminar* (Melbourne, Australia: 11 May 1985, forthcoming).

[5]*Diagnostic and Statistical Manual of Mental Disorders*, 3d ed. (Washington, D.C.: American Psychiatric Association, 1980), pp. 241-52; 285-90.

[6]J. Newmark, "Arm Difficulties Experienced by Musicians," Mind, Body, and the Performing Arts Conference, New York University, 18 July 1985.

[7]Richard Lederman, "A Medical Center for Performing Artists: Organization and Approach," International Conference of Symphony and Opera Musicians, San Francisco, California, 17 August 1985.

effect of making the teacher defensive and the pupil secretive. While the musician's technique is one of the three major factors in the equation of overuse, it is not the only one.

Overuse can occur in the great and famous as well as the aspiring student. The former are affected far more than is generally realized, including musicians possessing superlative technique so acknowledged by their peers. In other hand-use intensive occupations, the condition generally occurs when the work load goes up, the technique itself not altering. A teacher is expected to get a spectrum of results, and the students who try just as hard but who do not achieve quite what the better students accomplish are probably unfairly accused of "misuse." To handicapped people particularly, the meaning of this word is important, for it contains within its meaning an implication of abuse, of willful, improper use that is foreign to one's common experience with musicians and would be repugnant to the handicapped person. This is, at best, a misuse of the language.

The Present Study

This study came into being largely because of the difficulty in bridging the intellectual gap between the presentation of patients with music-related injuries and their commonly accepted explanations and supposed pathology. It was hoped that the study would reveal: (1) from what structures the pain was originating; (2) how the condition could be effectively treated; (3) how the condition could be prevented; and (4) how often it occurred, i.e., the incidence in musical populations.

The patients in the study came from three sources. The first group consisted of members of nine symphony orchestras. These musicians were interviewed and examined by the writer. In one orchestra, it was possible to examine only one-third of the members. In the remaining eight orchestras, however, virtually all the players were examined. The second group included the staff and students of nine tertiary music schools in Australia. The third group was comprised of private referrals--musicians who came to the writer for assessment and treatment.

Those with overuse injury were included in this series. The total number of people involved, at this writing, is over 650. Physical examination was restricted to those parts of the body directly or indirectly involved in the overuse process, and general examination was not carried out. Musicians seen with specific clinical conditions such as true tenosynovitis, nerve entrapments, etc., were excluded from the series. Though not

112

included in this series, references for tissue behavior were constantly made to patients in other occupations who had contracted the same condition. This was of great assistance in preventing any temptation to isolate the musicians from the rest of the community and ignore factors of commonality.

Results

The first 379 patients with overuse injury analyzed by tabulation showed the following results:

1. Age range was eight years to seventy years

2. Thirty percent of the patients could be classified as students, and there were two females for every male. The remaining 70% were performers, and within this group, there were two males for every female

3. All performance areas were affected: string players nearly 50%; woodwinds just over 20% keyboard nearly 20%; brass about 10%; and percussion, 4%

4. Concern increased with the length of time the condition had been present. Ten percent of the musicians had had their condition for more than ten years, and there was a peak incidence of two to five years' duration. Females between the ages of twelve to sixteen were the most vulnerable group

5. Pain was present in the hands and wrists in 50% of the patients, elsewhere in the upper limb in 30%. Fifty-five percent of the musicians complained of symptoms at least at one spinal level

6. Some attempt to grade the severity of the condition seemed imperative, however arbitrary this might seem. While the severity and extent of the physical signs (to be described later) were perhaps the most important factors, the length of history and the functional disablement were vital factors too. The injuries in this series seemed almost naturally to fall into five grades, as follows:

Grade 1 (30%) Pain is experienced in one site while playing the instrument. Pain stops when playing stops

Grade 2 (30%) Pain is felt in more than one site while playing, with a possible slight loss of coordination and loss of the very "top" of concert artist performance. Physical signs are either absent or minimal

Grade 3 (20%) Early involvement of painful hand use is experienced in activities other than making music. Pain persists when away from the instrument; physical signs are present; the student "under-performs," the orchestral player has a problem with the heavy work load; there may be a loss of response (speed, agility), a control (accuracy) representing loss of muscle function

Grade 4 (14%) Painful use of the hand is felt in all common social and domestic hand use, such as turning faucets on and off, unscrewing jar lids, writing, knitting, housework, typing, as well as music making. These tasks can still be carried out, though capacity is somewhat reduced, and pain is present. Students perform poorly; orchestral players adapt--in some instances--although some time off from work is common. There are marked physical signs of tissue damage and loss of muscle function

Grade 5 (6%) All uses of the hand are painful, and capacity is lost. The player's career is stopped or seriously threatened. Even the highly adaptive orchestral players have to cease performing. Students are unable to continue their programs. There are gross physical signs and continuous pain

Clinical Results--Symptoms

A symptom is something felt by the patient, such as pain or nausea. These symptoms cannot be measured nor displayed. In overuse injury, the predominating symptom is pain. In the upper limb, this may begin with a feeling of heaviness or tightness, discomfort, or even weakness. Sometimes there are pins and needles through the hands and fingers. These sensations are felt in the muscle groups, often in the forearm or shoulder, but frequently in the small muscles of the hand. The pain will tend to spread to other muscle groups nearby if the musician continues to play or practice. These symptoms may start while the musician is practicing, or they may begin some hours later, even the following day. The musician may complain of loss of strength and loss of coordination. In a few instances, loss of coordination may occur without pain. This development is clearly related to excessive use and is possibly due to "silent" muscle damage, perhaps akin to the "silent" coronary occlusion that occurs without pain.

Chronic fluctuating depression is usually present, but apart from this the personality of the musician is consistent with a normal and expected reaction to a disabling condition. As mentioned earlier, some of these patients were told that there was nothing the matter with them, and this information caused them to become more disturbed. The necessity for psychiatric referral was well under 5%.

Physical Signs

A physical sign is a demonstrable finding. A swelling anywhere on the body that can be measured and felt, and deformity of a bone due to fracture are good examples. Tenderness in a structure that is not normally tender is one of the most important signs in clinical surgery, despite the fact that it is partly subjective. The convincing demonstration of tenderness depends largely upon the non-verbal communication or "body language" and is usually unmistakable when this is demonstrated by an experienced surgeon. In this series, the structures found to have abnormal tenderness were the muscles (which are all doing the mechanical work) and joint ligaments that take the strain across the joint from one bone to another and are repetitively deformed in movement.

Muscle tissue becomes tender when it is injured either acutely or chronically. The ligaments of the joint behave in a similar way, becoming tender when they are damaged either from acute injury or from chronic overuse. Muscle biopsy studies are in progress.

The most marked physical signs are seen in tenderness of the intrinsic muscles of the hand in musicians who complain of painful hands and wrists. In addition to the instrinsic muscles being tender, the joint ligaments most affected are on the thumb side of the wrist (radial ligament) and the ligaments at the most basal joint of the thumb (the carpo-metacarpal joint). Where possible, the two hands should be examined simultaneously so that the registration of tenderness by body language is all the more convincing. This examination has been recorded in detail by the writer.[8] The extensor and flexor muscle groups of the forearm, and their common origin, the triceps muscle, the triceps insertion, the biceps, the muscles around the shoulder, particularly the rotator cuff and the scapula muscles, may all show tenderness. Tenderness of the neck muscles and the muscles along the spine may also be demonstrated, although in the case of spinal pain in musicians, a skeletal element is added to that of pure muscle overuse.

Two clarinetists, one trombonist, and one trumpet player were examined for loss of embouchure with accompanying pain in

---

[8]See footnote no. 2.

the facial muscles. In all these cases, tenderness of the damaged muscle matched up with pain in the area. Loss of function of the muscle of the palate was present in two oboists examined during this series. The function loss, however, was not examined at the time the muscle damage took place. Oboe players showing a dilation of the neck through stretching of the muscles of the throat did not appear to have tenderness. *The tenderness in the muscle and joint ligaments were often recorded years after the causal activity ceased* and were arbitrarily recorded 1 to 5 in degrees of severity.

In this series, there was one musician showing coincidental tenosynovitis of the deQuervain type.

Causal Activity

It appears to be continuous and intensive use, rather than the single episode or occasional use, that causes overuse injury as described here. During the recent MEH symposium, Richard Lederman (Cleveland Clinic) recognized the legitimate extension of overuse to include a single traumatic incident, "acute overuse."[9]

Most music making is carried out by repetitious activity of the hands and limbs, which implies some sort of relaxation phase in most of the muscle activity. Potentially more damaging, however, is the continuous muscle contraction from static loading. This not only increases the amount of muscle work that is carried out--there being no relaxation phase--but also increases the tensile load on the joint ligaments that transmit the weight across a joint from one bone to another. The B-flat clarinet (800 gms) and the oboe (about 600 gms), loaded on the right thumb, are good examples of needless and potentially highly damaging static loading on the thumb.

The joint at the base of the thumb suffers highly geared leverage, injuring the joint ligaments. In addition, the little muscles of the hand in the first cleft between the thumb and the side of the hand are kept in a state of tight contraction to maintain the relationship between the thumb and the rest of the hand. This muscular contraction is unremitting. The clarinetists' injuries (forty-nine in number) of this type are among the most frequent and severe in the series. One patient sustained an overuse injury in the left hand from carving oboe reeds. The right hand used the knife for carving, while the left hand held the reeds.

---

[9]Dr. Lederman made the remark during a roundtable discussion.

The trombone can produce this injury in the left hand, which is responsible for holding up the instrument. In the case of the string players, the bowing hand (right hand) sustained an overuse injury almost as often as the left hand (the fingering hand), although the injury to the left hand tended to be more serious.

The most uncompromising of all the static loading is possibly that suffered by the violinist and violist, where the instrument is held between the chin and the left shoulder. While there is intermittent and partial relief provided by the first cleft of the left hand, there is already evidence that holding up these instruments in this way is responsible for many symptoms of muscle overuse, hastening the degenerative procedures in the neck (cervical spondylosis) and shortening the player's performance life.

Intermediate Antecedents to Overuse

The most significant correlation in this series was that between student and performer and increase in playing and/or practice time. There was no reason to suppose that any radical change of technique occurred or that factors other than that of increased use of intensity and time were in operation.

The same phenomenon was noted in the case of potters who worked longer hours to prepare an exhibition and developed their overuse injury in this way.[10] The secretary suffering an overuse injury from a word processor sometimes did so at a time when an increased work load occurred. With musicians, the immediate precipitating factors were often a particular exercise, a new or difficult work, or an attempt to change technique (perhaps because of a new teacher). Students who had been away on vacation often began practicing hard without "easing in," and this frequently produced injuries. The music camp, while being one of the most enjoyable of the group music experiences, was associated with a high risk of injury due to the radically increased playing or practice time (sometimes quadrupled). Once again, the clarinetists are disproportionately represented.

The factor complex that correlates best with the onset of overuse injury appears to be the intensity of muscle use multiplied by the time involved.

---

[10]Fry, "Overuse Injury in Potters." See footnote on p. 2 of this text.

"Bad Teaching and Misuse"

These are allegations heard rather frequently. The allegation of bad teaching puts the responsibility of overuse injury on the teacher. The rationale is that the teacher is doing something wrong or teaching some faulty technique or offending some absolute standard of correctness. If this allegation is extended into studio conditions, the music teacher is asked to regard overuse injuries as "events that happen to somebody else's students." Should that teacher's own student contract an overuse injury, it is hardly surprising that the student may not wish to confide in the teacher.

The present study did not show evidence of teachers encouraging their students to excesses, at least as this applies in the situation of the Australian music schools involved. Errors of commission, as far as one can ascertain, did not show up as being a significant factor in the incidence of overuse injuries. A certain rigidity in approach, however, was noticed, and this did show up as a negative factor. For instance, in books on piano technique, points of difference rather than points of similarity were constantly stressed. Indeed, most such books are mutually exclusive in terms of "correctness."

While Horowitz, Ashkenazy, and Iturbi play with quite different techniques, there are simple and obvious common factors. All three performers avoid excessive uncoordinated muscular contractions, extreme positions, and awkward movements that require much more muscular effort and joint ligament loading.

There may be excessive muscular contraction on both sides of a joint, more than is required merely to stabilize it for the task at hand. Such excessive tension will mean that when quick movement is required, the joint will be less responsive and take more effort to move because of the existing muscular tension. Errors of omission on the part of the music teacher are, for the most part, due to inadequate briefing and direction from the medical profession. Music teachers are responsible for transmitting this wonderful element in our culture from one generation to the next. As one would expect from the nature of their task, they are, in the main, caring, compassionate educators who take their responsibility seriously. Music teachers can expect a spectrum of results reflected in the technique of their students.

Errors of omission come about largely through unavailability of medical information. There are three main matters of importance that are often defective because of this: (1) awareness of overuse injury; (2) questions of posture; and (3) practice habits.

118

While awareness of overuse injury may be a controversial matter, the dispute is a current one, and information is becoming more accessible to the music teacher. Of greatest importance is the notion that this is a preventable tragedy, and therefore it is essential that the music teacher learn as much as possible about the physical consequences of music making.

There are questions of posture. Included among these is the axiom that "the best spine is a straight spine;" preservation of a free range of movement of all joints; the necessity for a balanced set of physical activities for the musician (swimming is particularly good); and body awareness and control, as exemplified by Alexander, Feldenkrais, Yoga, and many other modes.

Practice habits should be *disciplined rather than dedicated*. Long hours of continuous music practice without breaks becomes mindless after a time, and the law of diminishing return operates as the risk of injury rises. Madsen and Madsen have shown that, in music tasks, the distraction rate rises significantly after about twenty-five minutes. If a five-minute break is then taken, concentration is restored for the next segment of twenty-five minutes. These workers found this to give the greatest value if effective and productive concentration is to be maintained.[11] There is an even more urgent reason, however, why such regular breaks in practice should be taken.

All of the body movement involved in practice is brought about by the contraction of muscles. They are a little like a car battery in that energy has been stored, and in muscular movement some of the stored energy is consumed. The blood flowing through muscles provides them with oxygen and glucose, which are the basic substances required to restore the energy to the system. During vigorous practice, restitution can not keep pace with usage. The muscle, therefore, goes into a state of debt for oxygen, among other things. Chemical restitution is very complex and occurs at various levels at different rates. It is really much more complicated than a car battery, although an analogy may be made. Damage may occur to the muscle in debt much as it occurs in the case of an improperly cared for car battery.

Twenty-five minutes is an adequate length of practice time. If a five-minute break is then taken, some restitution is possible, and even though the musician will not feel anything happening in the

---

[11]The research referred to was discussed with the writer by Clifford K. Madsen (The Florida State University) at the recent MEH symposium.

hands or arms, the changes that are occurring are complex and totally beneficial. At the end of the five-minute break, the musician will usually notice that the muscles are more responsive, especially if a new and difficult work is being learned. The practice then becomes more efficient and effective if such regular breaks are taken. Practice segments should be shorter for small children who are gifted.

In addition to the above factors, the music student who practices ten to twelve hours a day is isolated from the rest of the community. In the interests of a balanced education, excessively long hours of practice should not be encouraged.

"Misuse"

This term is often applied to the less skillful, less coordinated player using excessive muscular activity. The term, however, implies an active, willful, and purposely harmful type of use--more like a punishable offense! The inescapable implication is that it is the student's fault, and once having decided this, true inquiry ceases. This is unlikely to give the student any confidence, for there are two other factors in the overuse equation in addition to technique.

Three Factors in Overuse Injury

The three factors in overuse injury are: (1) genes; (2) musical technique; and (3) intensity multiplied by the time of playing.

Genes

Every individual is a "genetic once off," being the product of millions of generations of such individual ancestors who have gone before. Individuals are known to have certain capabilities in physical performance or endurance that are constantly being put to the test in competition. Variable vulnerability to overuse injury would automatically follow from this. If the product of intensity of use multiplied by time is a theoretical notion that can be accepted, then the time that the individual exceeds his own specifications in this regard becomes defined when there is resulting damage in the working tissues. While the other two factors are, of course, also operating, there appears to be a certain genetic "pecking order."

The individuals who are less robust genetically will suffer overuse before those who have a higher threshold because of

120

greater *capacity* for "intensity multiplied by time." When one is dealing with large numbers of individuals, the other two factors will even out. A good example of this is the clarinet student practicing about an hour and a quarter a day, loading the eight hundred gram clarinet on the right thumb. When such a student goes to music camp, this time may be quadrupled. Factor three (intensity multiplied by time) then becomes almost a fixed quantity, the only other variable being factor two (technique). If techniques are examined closely, there is usually not a wide variety of difference within a group. It has also been shown that the main damaging factor in clarinet playing is the static loading on the right thumb. Under these circumstances, the genetically less robust people will suffer injury first and, during a period of about three weeks at a music camp, individuals will suffer injury in a certain order because of their genetically determined vulnerability to break down.

The Technique

Musical technique is the exclusive province of the music teacher, not the medical doctor. The music teacher employs the skills and experience to encourage the student in an energy-use efficient means of playing the instrument. Excessive and uncoordinated muscular contraction is discouraged so that joints are stabilized with the minimum amount of muscular use that is maximally coordinated. It is easy to see that if any joint used during music making is stabilized by excessive muscular pull on both sides, the result will be that the joint will be less responsive when executant muscle contraction occurs. In addition, such muscle contraction has to be more forceful to move the joint that is stabilized by such excessive muscular pull. It is also self-evident that such a student will not be performing maximally well using this type of muscular activity. A student or, indeed, a performer who uses the more effortless coordinated technique will always be further away from the threshold of overuse injury than the student or performer who employs the more tense technique described above.

A parallel may be perceived in the common act of writing. Most people write with excessive muscular force. Once the end joint of the index finger of the writing hand is hyper-extended (over-straightened), one must remember that the muscle carrying out this action is located high up in the forearm and must be balanced by an equal amount of forceful contraction on the other side of the forearm, since these muscles cross both the wrist and the elbow joints. This uncoordinated muscular contraction tends to spread and, in extreme cases, involves not only the upper arm but the shoulder and neck as well. Based on an educated guess of the muscle mass involved in this writing style (using more muscle mass than necessary), it may take the person as much as one hundred times the amount of muscle tissues to write in this way than is strictly necessary. Since writing is also the cause of overuse injury, retraining has to take place here too.

Intensity and time

Available evidence suggests that no matter how genetically robust any given musician may be, he will suffer overuse injury if he plays long enough and/or intensely enough. This is based on the proposition that there is an upper level of tolerance that must exist even though it cannot be defined until breakdown occurs. Since all body tissues and, indeed, all known materials do have an upper level tolerance, this proposition would appear to hold true.

This is supported by the music camp example of the clarinetists who increase drastically their practice or playing time over a three-week period. Injuries that occur are directly attributable to the static loading of a clarinet on the right thumb. It seems to be a "dose dependent" breakdown. A logical extension of this situation would be to imagine (perhaps absurdly) the same young people practicing perhaps fourteen hours a day and continuing on for long enough until all players had been affected. The writer has actually seen an example of heavy rehearsal of an advanced primary school orchestra where all six clarinetists became progressively affected, except for one who supported the clarinet with a post and was, therefore, not loaded on the right thumb.

It must be accepted, therefore, that this proposition of an upper limit in all musicians must be there and that it is sensible to respect it rather than to define it. Doing otherwise involves the risk of overuse injury.

Previous Treatment

Approximately one-quarter of the patients in this series with muscular and joint capsule overuse had been treated with anti-inflammatory drugs. They reported no significant help but a very high incidence of side effects. These musicians did not believe that the course of their condition was significantly altered, though some noted a little short-term diminution of pain. While one may postulate that the injury would lead to the production of degradation products that have an inflammatory effect, such results would be secondary.

Similarly, muscle relaxants and other drugs were, in the main, unhelpful in terms of any significant effect on the cause of the condition. Those who continued to practice or play invariably became worse. In particular, patients who had alternative splinting and exercises suffered an increase in their pain, and in this series one could find no evidence that this benefited the course of their condition. Musicians who were given complete rest from playing reported variable relief.

In the first 379 musicians with overuse injury in this series, operative treatment had been carried out as follows: six patients had carpal tunnel operations; seven had tenosynovectomies on the extensor tendon sheath; two had ulnar nerve transposition; two had resection of the first rib; and two had two operations each for decompression of the posterior interosseous nerve. None of these procedures relieved the underlying condition.

While musicians, like any other part of the population, may contract nerve entrapment syndromes, it seemed that these results showed that overuse did mimic true nerve entrapments and that this clearly was a potential for inaccuracy.

Potential Treatment in the Present Series

For Grade 1, 2, and certain kinds of Grade 3 overuse injuries, the appropriate approach would appear to be a collection of supportive measures. Some important measures include: clinical examination of the musician's technique to improve energy-use efficiency, review of repertoire, improvement of posture, exercises to improve range of movement of spinal and other joints, and attention to general health. Body awareness and control may be taught in various ways--through Alexander, Feldenkrais, Yoga, and other techniques.

It is important to remove static loading of heavy instruments. One cannot stress too much the importance of avoiding this useless and potentially damaging, counter-productive muscular use. Practice habits must be disciplined rather than dedicated. Hour after hour of practice without breaks should be discouraged. It is far better to practice in segments of around twenty-five minutes with a five-minute break *by the clock.* The muscles will be more responsive and less drained by this. Some absolute upper limit of practice should be agreed upon, and gradual elevation of practice load should be adopted.

In the case of Grade 4, 5, and most Grade 3 injuries, rest appears to be the only means likely to give substantial help if the above measures have failed or, if when first seen, the musician presents one of the more serious examples of physical injury. Other studies, such as Lederman's at the Cleveland Clinic, Hochberg and Leffert at Massachussetts General, and Schneck at the Denver Musicians Clinic, are agreed on an adequate period of rest in order to heal the injury.

The first aim of treatment is to render the musician pain free, and the second is to return him to the instrument. The longer the symptoms and signs have been present, the longer the "healing" process will take. The resolution of symptoms and signs is, in the writer's opinion, the proper criterion for healing and, therefore, the signal that the musician is ready to go back to music making.

Radical rest is required. Grades 3 to 5 injuries experience pain in the hands or wrists (or elsewhere), and aggravating activities, in addition to playing, must be stopped as well. Ongoing pain probably means ongoing damage, and experience with the series indicated that while these activities were carried out, the injuries persisted and in some instances even became worse. Activities such as driving, writing, food preparation, and housework should not be carried out in a program of *total avoidance of pain-inducing activities*. This means help in the house, explanation to and organization of other family members, cooperation from the employer or music school, and, generally, a support system to allow such a program of rest to be properly carried out.

Total avoidance of pain-inducing activities does not involve the use of drugs unless pain at night is distressing, in which case aspirin may initially be used. Splints are not required unless pain interferes with sleep or the patient wakes with pain due to the posture of the wrist on waking, e.g., full downward flexion.

In the first two to three weeks, the pains increase, often become sharper in quality, and arise from new areas. In addition, the fluctuating depression usually becomes worse before it gets better. This early response to the treatment is discouraging, and support from the physician is required by weekly appointments. This course of events must be explained in advance if the patient is to stay on the program. Sometimes this bad period may be prolonged.

After this time, the symptoms and signs wax and wane, and the musician who stays with the program gradually experiences freedom from pain and signs. This may take up to six months, occasionally longer. Fortunately, in some instances, the time is shorter. Practice of the instrument should be resumed infinitely gradually, starting with perhaps two minutes twice a day, and working up to two minutes in the hour. Even this amount may cause aching in the unused muscles to begin with. In this case, a day or two away from the instrument may be needed after this first try. Very gradually and *by the clock,* the musician works up to perhaps twenty minutes in each hour, very gradually increasing the intensity of practice.

Many musicians express initial concern that their unused muscles will wither and will never recover their previous capacity or skills. Fortunately, one can assure the musicians that this is not the case. While the muscles do revert to a more baseline condition in terms of capacity, the experience with the program so far indicates that the skills are retrievable and that the muscles do not atrophy (wither).

Incidence

The incidence of injuries both in music schools and orchestras is an index of the importance of this matter.

Music Schools

In this study, which included seven out of Australia's ten performance schools, the mean incidence was 9.3%.[12] This was a bedrock figure as other overuse injuries were known to have occurred.In one music school serviced by clinics, the incidence was 21%, and although it should be stressed that many of these injuries were not serious, the incidence does give cause for concern. Since the evidence from this study indicates that injuries will get worse rather than better unless something is done about them, the early reporting of injuries is going to reduce ultimate disablement and "drop out."

The Symphony Orchestra

At the time of writing, nine symphony orchestras had been examined and those players with overuse subjected to physical examination. All orchestras showed an incidence of greater than 50% of overuse incidence injury, and even when Grade 1 injuries

---

[12]Hunter J. H. Fry, "The Prevalence of Overuse [Injury] Syndrome in Australian Music Schools, *British Journal of Industrial Medicine,* in press.

were excluded, the incidence did not fall below 30% in any of the orchestras and remained as high as 50% at the other end of the scale.[13]

This evidence is very suggestive that this is a "carry on" phenomenon from the music school and gives considerable cause for concern. There must be few occupations where the occurrence of occupational pain is as common as this.

The Overuse Concept

All living tissues work within relatively fine tolerances, and if the upper tolerance is exceeded, damage will occur. Excessive sound will damage the internal ear, excessive light will damage the eye, excessive force will fracture the bone, and excessive tension will break the skin. Muscle tissue is damaged by excessive use and contraction. Howard in 1937 and Thompson et al. in 1951 demonstrated muscular damage in workers carrying out repetitious factory work.[14] This also occurs in "iron pumpers" who damage their muscles with excessive body building exercises. Some victims of poliomyelitis have muscles that are already overperforming. These people suffer overuse when they undergo increased physical activity. Joint ligaments are pain sensitive structures and become painful if they are injured either from acute or chronic overuse. In acute overuse (the sprained ankle), such a torn ligament is exceedingly tender and in damage from chronic use. The ligaments are usually permanently swollen (often referred to as "peri-articular swelling").

While the whole upper limb is involved in most music making, the hands are of special interest. The intrinsic muscles of the hand flex the first bone of the finger on the hand and also spread the fingers and are, therefore, responsible for positioning and moving the fingertips. In an extended practice session, these muscles may ache, but the ache soon goes. It has been observed that in intensive use of the hands, the pain from overuse may not

---

[13]Hunter J. H. Fry, "The Incidence of Overuse Injury Syndrome in the Symphony Orchestra Medical Problems of Performing Artists," in press.

[14]N. J. Howard, "Peritendinitis Crepitans," *Journal of Bone and Joint Surgery* 19 (April 1937):447-59; A. R. Thompson, L. W. Plewes, and E. G. Shaw, "Peritendinitis Crepitans and Simple Tenosynovitis: A Clinical Study of 544 Cases in Industry," *British Journal of Industrial Medicine* 8 (1951):150-60.

immediately appear after excessive use but rather occurs a variable time *after* the causal activity. In acute use, by contrast, the onset of pain usually prevents muscular overuse.

It was interesting to notice that in the other occupations affected by overuse injury, when one limb was affected, it was the limb that worked the harder, not necessarily the dominant side.

Prevention

The prevention of overuse is the control of use. In the case of the musician, there are four factors that appear to matter: (1) music practice; (2) static loading; (3) education of music students; and (4) general health.

1. Muscle is a remarkable tissue, having the high level of stored energy that, at will, can be transformed into mechanical energy. Unless adequate rest periods are taken, however, healthy restitution is not possible. Imagine the "reductio ad absurdum" of a musician practicing say sixteen hours a day, where the remaining eight hours are simply insufficient to allow the chemical changes involved in muscle restitution to take place. For reasons explained above, a twenty-five minute practice segment followed by a five minute break is a very reasonable baseline scheme, not only for muscle and joint ligament health, but also to allow physical and mental tension to dissipate and for the concentration span to be restored

2. Holding up an instrument is a significant factor in the production of overuse injury when the playing or practice load is high. This applies to the right thumb (clarinet), the French horn (arms and spine), or the violin (neck and left shoulder). The act of holding up the instrument is a totally useless, non-productive, energy expenditure that reduces responsiveness of the involved joints that require greater force to move them. A young child learning to play the clarinet who begins playing with a post (so that the clarinet is weightless) will not suffer overuse injury and will advance more rapidly in technique. The same general argument applies to other instruments

3. Unless the facts about overuse are known to students, they remain unprotected and highly vulnerable because of their dedication. Most music students do not understand the difference between dedicated practice, which represents long hours of application, and disciplined practice of the type described above, where the student has to stop playing when he may not feel like doing so. If students in music schools are taught the nature of

overuse injury, its consequences, and, above all, its prevention, they will be given the type of protection that will enable them to make good decisions when they are in the practice room.

4. The writer's own observations would clearly indicate that the student survives the vicissitudes of late adolescence much better if care is taken of the general health. Most music students do not know how the body works, the essential cyclic nature of our existence, and the necessity for certain baseline regularities. The body easily accepts acute variations, but less easily accepts chronic variations. Overuse injuries in the spine are common among musicians. They should be taught about good posture and that "the best spine is a straight spine." In addition, they need to know that early development of the best set of muscles to support the spine is important. Body awareness and control, by whatever system it is taught, can only be beneficial

These questions of education ought, in my view, to be examinable material in the music schools, particularly those that are the main suppliers of professional musicians who perform in orchestras, chamber ensembles, and as soloists.

Conclusions

1. *Stop when it hurts!* Pain in the hands and arms is a danger signal, not an achievement. The doctrine of "practice until it hurts" is dangerous. While many students survive such habits, others do not, and this represents excessive zeal and dedication that is *potentially self-destructive*

2. Where there is severe overuse injury, the musician should not be returned to the instrument until the symptoms and signs have settled. In premature resumption of music practice, the condition will probably recur, leading to mental as well as physical trauma. Again, there will be those musicians who will "get away with it," but this is taking a gamble that, in a "one career" individual, is probably not acceptable

3. The program of total avoidance of pain-inducing activities (T.A.P.I.A.) needs a great deal of organization and support. It is not a simple matter and, if treated as such, will not work. This is highly demanding of the physician as well as of the patient. The program should not be entered into lightly. It is probably the safest treatment that one can imagine, since there are no operations, no drugs, and no use of damaged structures until they are ready for it

4. Musicians may contract surgically treated conditions, like any other group in the community. Pain originating from damaged muscles and ligaments tends to have a rather odd type of pain radiation. "Pins and needles," suggesting nerve involvement, is not uncommon. Various observations would suggest that pharmacologically active substances are produced in overuse that further complicate the picture. Strict criteria should be maintained for surgical intervention in the case of nerve entrapment syndromes. In the case of the highly contentious thoracic outlet syndrome, the only criterion that really matters is the result

5. Musicians contracting overuse injury do not really want to stop playing if this can be avoided. The physician is therefore tempted to advise them to continue to play, but to treat them with anti-inflammatory drugs that, from the observations in this series, do not alter the basic course of the disease. In severe examples of overuse, this will lead to further trouble

6. Disciplined rather than dedicated practice is more logical for the hard-working muscular structures and the joint ligaments taking the loading. Removing the static load from the weight of the instrument will further reduce muscular work and bring about an improvement in technique. These two positive factors increase the efficiency of music making while decreasing the load

REFERENCES

Browne, C. D.; Nolan, B. M.; and Faithfull, D. K. "Occupational Repetition Strain Injuries: Guidelines for Diagnosis and Management." *Medical Journal of Australia* 140 (March 1984):329-32.

Diagnostic and Statistical Manual of Mental Disorders. 3d ed. Washington, D.C.: American Psychiatric Association, 1980.

Fry, Hunter J. H., "The Incidence of Overuse Injury Syndrome in the Symphony Orchestra Medical Problems of Performing Artists." In press.

_____. "Occupational Maladies of Musicians: Their Cause and Prevention." *International Journal of Music Education* 2 (November 1984):63-66.

_____. "Overuse Injury in Potters." *Pottery in Australia* 24, no. 3 (September 1985):48.

_____. "Overuse Injury Syndrome in the Upper Limb in Musicians." *Medical Journal of Australia,* in press.

_____. "Physical Signs in the Hand and Wrist Seen in the Overuse Injury Syndrome of the Upper Limb." *Australian and New Zealand Journal of Surgery,* in press.

_____. "The Prevalence of Overuse [Injury] Syndrome in Australian Music Schools." *British Journal of Industrial Medicine.* In press.

Howard, N. J. "Peritendinitis Crepitans." *Journal of Bone and Joint Surgery* 19 (April 1937): 447-59.

Kimber, W. "R.S.I. and Musicians." *Victoria Ministry of Arts Seminar.* Melbourne, Australia: Ministry of Arts. forthcoming.

Lederman, Richard. "A Medical Center for Performing Artists: Organization and Approach." Paper presented at the International Conference of Symphony and Opera Musicians, San Francisco, California, 17 August 1985.

Newmark, J. "Arm Difficulties Experienced by Musicians." Paper presented at the Mind, Body, and the Performing Arts Conference, New York University, 18 July 1985.

Thompson, A. R.; Plewes, L. W.; and Shaw, E. G. "Peritendinitis Crepitans and Simple Tenosynovitis: A Clinical Study of 544 Cases in Industry." *British Journal of Industrial Medicine* 8 (1951):150-60.

HUMAN WELL-BEING OF VISUALLY IMPAIRED STUDENTS THROUGH ACCOMMODATION IN MUSIC CLASSES FOR THE SIGHTED

by

FRED KERSTEN

The Changing Scene

Public Laws 93-112 and 94-142 have provided impetus for including handicapped individuals in public school and higher education programs. Although now in effect for other disabilities, the process of "mainstreaming" actually began around 1960 for the visually impaired. At that time, just about half of these students were in residential schools--an increase of 41% from 1950. Lowenfeld (1975) has verified these enrollment statistics for blind children in residential and day schools during 1950, 1960, and 1972.

By 1972, 68.5% of those considered blind were enrolled in day school classes. A letter received in 1978 from the New York State Department of Social Services indicated that more that 1600 (80%) of approximately 2000 elementary and high school blind students are currently attending public schools. Kersten (1979) conducted a recent survey of residential schools for the blind and found that two of these schools had closed their doors because of the mainstreaming trend, while other schools were moving toward serving students whose multihandicaps required institutionalization.

Visually impaired people who enter sighted persons' environments are encouraged to become involved in music programs. Participation is important to visually impaired people because: (a) music is helpful physiologically, providing relaxation to fatigued aural senses that substitute for lack of sight; (b) music provides aesthetic experience in a world that can become barren and dreary; and (c) music allows for a degree of physiological and psychological equivalency with the sighted, a vital aspect of the self-image and esteem needs of nonsighted individuals.

Music educators with limited training in teaching visually impaired students are sometimes hesitant about including these individuals in their programs. Such reluctance may be due to lack of familiarity with: (a) teaching methodology, (b) audio-mechanical aids, and (c) instructional resources that can be used to accommodate these persons effectively in music classrooms. This paper will provide practical suggestions for instruction and describe materials and procurement sources for music educators whose classes include visually impaired persons. New technological developments designed to facilitate learning in the future will also be examined.

Classroom Accommodation

There are many references in the literature to teachers who, through a mistaken sense of kindness and solicitude, project an impression of pity. Visually impaired people hate the word pity! Coates (1976) advises teachers how to avoid this problem:

> Don't feel sorry for your blind students and don't try to be overly helpful. If a blind person is to function and to live his own life to the fullest, he must learn to get by on his own, and he must never indulge in self-pity or allow himself to become overly dependent on others. (p. 29)

Coates also indicated that it is perfectly natural for teachers to refer to color of piano keys and use such words as "see" and "look." Avoidance can only cause an awkward, self-conscious situation.

"Psychological problems of blindness are more in the minds of others rather than in the blind themselves" (Freedman, 1975, p. 10). Students and teachers can facilitate an effective music education only if they understand what visually impaired people can and cannot do.

First, there should be an investigation of the specific dynamics of each person's disability. Severity of individual handicaps must be an important first discovery. Many so-called blind individuals have varied amounts of residual sight that can be effectively used to read large-print scores, without resorting to braille music or audio devices for musical instruction. The writer made the mistake of teaching a piano student totally by rote and audio equipment, when large-print music could have been effectively used.

Classroom accommodation of visually impaired persons requires alteration of classroom management, instructional techniques, and musical considerations. The following suggestions are offered:

Classroom Management

1. Identify texts and music in advance and consult the National Library Service to see if large-print, audio, or braille copies are in existence. If not, transcriptions will have to be produced.

2. Orient students to the classroom and make sure that any changes in furniture arrangement are made known immediately. Doors or cupboards left partly open are particularly hazardous. Obstacles in hallways, such as drinking fountains, should be identified.

3. If you have to lead a visually impaired student, the proper and recommended technique is to have the person place one hand on your arm (near the elbow) and follow beside and slightly behind you.

4. Assign a sighted student to be responsible for leading the visually impaired person from the building in case a situation arises in which emergency egress is necessary.

5. The presence in the classroom of a guide dog will necessitate altered seating arrangements. A reserved seat near the door is recommended. Guide dogs are working dogs and should not become objects for affection. These animals have limitations and can be distracted from their duties.

Instructional Techniques

1. Record assignment information on cassette for those persons who cannot take notes on a braille slate.

2. Identify yourself when you enter the music room and announce when you are leaving.

3. Allow visually impaired students to participate musically whenever possible. Inclusion of these students in ensemble activities is mandatory in public schools. Participation in movement activities (as part of the general music class) can be achieved by providing the visually impaired person with a sighted partner and an unobstructed space.

4. Play aloud all musical examples written on the chalkboard or included within a text.

5. Expect reasonable standards of musical performance and academic achievement from visually impaired students. Realize that while the average college student reads at a rate of 500-800 words per minute (wpm) the braille user reads at about 60-80 wpm and, if audio aids are used, listens at 180-200 wpm. This means that reading assignments should be made well in advance of class sessions.

Musical Considerations

1. In an instrumental or choral ensemble, place visually impaired persons near a competent performer playing the same part. Many visually impaired people find that sitting in front of their section enables them to distinguish their part in addition to helping the ensemble with intonation and part memorization.

2. Entrances by nonsighted players are usually anticipated by listening for intake of breath by sighted peers. The timing between breath intake and group sound production serves as a cue for the visually impaired musician to begin.

3. Valved brass players and vocalists can read braille and perform simultaneously. Reading skills provide an added dimension to the performance of these individuals. Although prior preparation is necessary, it is important to minimize the memorization of lengthy band and choral compositions.

4. Visually impaired players do not realize an increase in musical aptitude or musicality because of sight loss. In the early 1900s, visually impaired individuals were thought to have a musical advantage and were encouraged to pursue music as a vocation. A professional musical career should be given careful consideration since problems of memorization and sightreading hinder even those with exceptional ability.

5. Students unable to use large-print notation who are contemplating careers in music must learn the braille system. While it is possible for repertoire to be taught by rote or audio means, the process of correcting mistakes or pieces already memorized and learning new music quickly becomes impossible without braille. The instructor who has identified those students with skills of professional caliber should immediately arrange for instruction in musical braille from local teachers. (Consult special service divisions within the state in order to find these teachers.) It is easier to teach musical braille to the young student. It is recommended that musical braille be taught when the student of about ten to twelve years of age, after a knowledge of literary braille has been developed.

6. It is not necessary for instructors to learn braille notation, although a general familiarity with it can be helpful in understanding what students perceive. An excellent book, *How to Read Braille Music,* by Bettye Krolick, can be obtained from the Stipes Publishing Company, Champaign,Illinois. Clearly illustrated, this short volume provides a basic understanding of the system within a few hours of study.

7. Melodic and rhythmic dictation can be notated in braille by visually impaired theory students. Instructors who need to determine if notation written in braille is correct will have to consult an expert. One solution to the problem is to have two cassette tape recorders. As students listen to recorded examples on one machine, they can verbally analyze what is heard and simultaneously record both the analysis and example on the second machine. Upon listening to the second tape, the instructor will be able immediately to tell if the answers are correct. Both methods of response should be encouraged. There should be a periodic checking of the braille symbols because a symbolic illiteracy can result if audio aids become the prevalent method of assessment.

8. It is easier for a student taking harmonic dictation to notate each musical line separately. The braille system requires additional signs for inner voices, and more symbols lead to complexity and, ultimately, confusion.

9. Visually impaired students can conduct and should be encouraged to do so. Sighted students may demonstrate various patterns by guiding visually impaired students' hands and arms. Raised line drawings will illustrate the "Gestalt" of each pattern and promote conceptual understanding. The instructor must watch for awkward habits and incorrect patterns and correct these immediately.

Variety of Available Musical Materials

Currently available musical materials have been developed over the years according to individual necessity and request. Large-print and braille copies have been produced as the need arose. An examination of material catalogs shows some interesting gaps in continuity. For example, it is possible to obtain a brailled second trumpet part for a band method and find that the first and/or third parts are unavailable. The specific part that is needed for a particular situation is the only part that is transcribed.

Series Books

Many general music series books in braille are available. A partial listing includes:

Silver Burdett Series
>*Making Music Your Own*
>*Music* (words only)
>*Music of Our Time* (text)

Birchard Music Series
>Grade 7
>Grade 8

Ginn Music Series
>*Singing and Rhyming* (words only)
>*Singing Every Day* (words only)
>*Singing in Harmony* (words only)
>*Singing Juniors* (words only)
>*Singing on Our Way* (words only)
>*The Magic of Music* (Books 2-6)

Holt, Rinehart, & Winston Series
>*Exploring Music* (text only)

Instrumental

Woodwind and brass players will find instructional materials that range from the *Arban Method* and *Art of French Horn Playing* to *Breeze-Easy* and *Rubank* beginners' books. Clarinetists may obtain copies of *Klose,* and saxophonists have the *Vereecken Foundation to Saxophone Playing.*

Percussionists can order *The American Drummer, Harr Drum Method,* and most beginning books. Music for strings dominates the catalogs. Violin, cello, and guitar occupy ranking positions with little or nothing available for viola or double bass. Concertos by Vivaldi, Mozart, and Paganini can be obtained for violinists, while the *Six Suites for Unaccompanied Cello* of J. S. Bach are available for cellists.

Piano

There is much brailled music available for piano. Fifty percent of the *American Printing House Catalog* is devoted to piano literature. Most standard and popular works are brailled for this medium. An increasing amount of large-print music can also be procured.

Band and Orchestra

There was a time when bands dominated music programs in residential schools for the blind. Therefore, full-band transcriptions brailled for these organizations are still available. There are also available transcriptions for orchestra. However, much of the material is extremely dated, and few contemporary compositions are represented. Today's ensemble director must plan on either braille or large-print transcription for a visually impaired person in the group.

Music for Voice

There is a substantial amount of transcribed music for choral ensemble. Most well-known choral pieces from oratorios, cantatas, operas, and musicals are available. There is also a great deal of solo literature.

Organ

A great amount of classical and popular organ music is available in transcribed form. The availability of this music is due to two factors: (a) There are vocational possibilities for church musicians and night club artists, and (b) visually impaired beginners can easily achieve satisfying musical results on modern electronic instruments. In addition, classical music transcribed for blind organists in France has found its way into American libraries, thereby augmenting the archives of available material.

Procuring Musical Materials

There are several organizations that may be contacted to obtain either copies or transcriptions services for visually impaired individuals. Braille, large-print, and recorded formats are usually available.

National Library Service (NLS) for the Blind and Physically Handicapped

The NLS is located in Washington, D.C. The library acts as a national repository and receives copies of materials transcribed by other sources. The NLS provides the most complete collection of resources in this country and probably in the world. Twenty-four thousand compositions make up the braille music collection.

Categories of musical materials represented include: braille music books; recorded aids for braille music; tape and disc recordings; bold note music; cassettes; and musical periodicals in braille, large print, and cassette format (Coates, 1976). *The Musical Mainstream* (1978), an NLS publication, provides a detailed description of specific materials and services obtainable from the NLS. The items include:

1. Braille books about music.
2. Braille music scores for all instruments and voice.
3. Beginning self-instruction courses on cassette for piano, organ, and guitar.
4. Cassette and disc copies of books, lectures, interviews, demonstrations, and other educational materials.
5. Large-print music scores for all instruments and voice.
6. Large-print books on music.
7. Talking-book disc subscriptions to *Stereo Review* and *Music Journal*.
8. *Contemporary Sound Track: A Review of Pop, Jazz, Rock, and Country.* Selected articles from print music and news periodicals, recorded on cassette.
9. *Popular Music Lead Sheets.* Braille transcriptions of words, melodies, and chords for selected old and new popular songs.
10. *Music Article Guide.* An annotated index to selected articles in about two hundred magazines in braille. Cassette copies of articles are supplied on demand. Reference services and assistance in locating information about music and musicians. (p. 69)

138

Musical Mainstream contains: reprints in large print of selected articles on music from major magazines, a listing of newly transcribed music, and an excellent column on braille music notation by Bettye Krolick. In addition to this resource, there are various available catalogs of materials, such as: *Music and Musicians--Instructional Cassette Recording Catalog, Music and Musicians--Instructional Disc Recording Catalog,* and *Braille Books about Music and Musicians.* Requests for materials should be sent to: Library of Congress, National Library Service for the Blind and Physically Handicapped, Washington, D. C. 20542.

Johanna Bureau for the Blind and Visually Handicapped Inc.

The Johanna Bureau, located at 30 West Washington Street, Chicago, Illinois, provides a library of resources and a transcription service. The *Johanna Music Catalog* (1978) is comprehensive and includes both classical and popular music.

Volunteer Services for the Blind (VSB)

Although Volunteer Services does not specialize in production of music, they do produce special-order books for students and professional people. Therefore, musical texts are available from this source. In addition, Recorded Periodicals, a division of VSB, produces recorded periodicals using the 15/16 ips cassette format. Recorded Periodicals is located at 919 Walnut Street, Philadelphia, Pennsylvania.

Hadley School for the Blind

The Hadley School at 700 Elm Street, Winnetka, Illinois, produces one musical publication, *How to Read Braille Music Notation,* available in correspondance course format.

National Braille Press, Inc.

Started in 1953, National Braille Press produces braille for individuals all over the world. The organization specializes in both literary and music materials. Darling (1965, p. 8) indicates that in the 1953-63 period, 19,335 pages of brailled music were produced by National Braille Press volunteers. National Braille Press is located at 88 St. Stephen Street, Boston, Massachussetts.

Recording for the Blind (RFB)

RFB provides facilities for recording books as requested by individuals. Music texts that have been recorded as part of the RFB library are available on loan at no charge. *A Catalog of Tape Recorded Books* may be requested from the RFB offices, located at 215 East 58th Street, New York, New York. RFB has an extensive collection of master volumes available. As of April 1974, 23,000 titles were available in the library, with an average increase of 350 newly recorded titles each month. The *RFB Catalog* numbers 1,127 pages. Borrowers must send in two copies of each book to be recorded because every recording is simultaneously proofread by a monitor. RFB services may be of value to musicology or music history professors who have visually impaired persons in their classes.

National Braille Association, Inc. (NBA)

NBA is a national organization of persons who are interested in developing and distributing materials to the visually impaired in America. Membership consists of individuals working in a volunteer capacity to produce braille transcriptions. The NBA address for memberships is: 654-A Godwin Avenue, Midland Park, New Jersey. The Braille Book Bank (BBB), sponsored by the NBA, is located in Rochester, New York at 422 Clinton Avenue. The Braille Book Bank provides transcriptions upon request.

The Braille Book Bank is nonprofit since costs are supported with money obtained from NBA. Book costs to students are thereby reduced. Established in 1963, BBB provides textbooks for high school and college students at an average rate of 300,000 braille pages a year.

The BBB Music Catalog lists originals that have been transcribed into braille and are obtainable as thermoform duplicates. The Table of Contents lists the following categories: General Works, Music Charts, Harmony, Theory, Piano, Organ, Stringed Instruments, Woodwinds, Brass, Percussion, Miscellaneous Instruments, Vocal and Chorus (1978-1979, p. x). Resources for guitar and piano are substantial, but limited for woodwinds. Most of the music in this catalog is classical.

American Printing House for the Blind (APH)

American Printing House for the Blind is the largest publisher for the blind in the world. It produces about one-half the world's press-printed braille, talking books (recordings), and large-type literature for the partially sighted. (*The World Book Encyclopedia*, 1974, vol. 1, p. 405.)

APH has been in existence since 1858 and its comprehensive production capacity makes its catalogs an important source for anyone contemplating purchase of a musical composition in braille. Two catalogs and supplements will be sent upon request.

The *Catalog of Music Publications* (1970), including the 1971-73 supplements, provides a guide to all types of musical materials. A Table of Contents for the 1970 catalog lists the following categories: Harmony; General Works; Music Notation; Piano Tuning; Piano--Grade 1 only; Piano Music; Vocal Music; Chorus Music for Mixed Voices; Organ Music; Stringed Instruments--Cello, Guitar, String Ensemble, Violin; Accordian Music; Brass and Wind Instruments; Band and Orchestra Music (1970, p. ii). Most of the music listed in the APH catalogs is classical; no popular or jazz music seems to have been transcribed into braille by the APH.

A second APH catalog, *1970 Music Selections Formerly Available from the Illinois Braille and Sight Saving School, Jacksonville, Illinois,* lists compositions produced by the print shop of the Illinois school when it was in operation. The collection, acquired by APH, includes works that have composition dates predominantly in the early 1900s. With the exception of a classified band music section, the Table of Contents is quite similar to the *APH Catalog.*

Sigma Alpha Iota

This national music fraternity has been significant in providing braille and large-print transcriptions. Information on volunteer music transcription services may be obtained by contacting the National Executive Office located at 4119 Rollins Avenue, Des Moines, Iowa 50312.

Audio-Mechanical Instruction

Through the years, attempts have been made to develop tactile devices to aid in the perception of notation patterns. Early, crude attempts at such devices are mentioned in the *Code de musique pratique,* by Jean Philippe Rameau (1760). One of these devices utilized metal and wooden type for physical notational representation.

Reuss (1935) mentions an attempt by Marie Therese von Paradis, the blind composer, to write down pieces utilizing a table she invented. This event took place while she was at the Court of Marie Antoinette. Unfortunately, this table failed since "she was unable to read her own compositions or to transcribe other musical compositions with the device" (p. 6).

Beetz Notation Graph

The Beetz Notation Graph has become a very popular device for instruction of staff notation. The notation graph allows students to "see" staff notation with their fingers. Hoy (1954) gives the following description of the device:

> The apparatus consists of a cork base upon which the staff lines and clefs are mounted. All other symbols used in music notation are supplied with the set and may be fastened upon the staves at will. The staff and all the symbols are made of wire to which pins have been soldered. (p. 51)

The Beetz Graph is important because it allows each student to develop an understanding of graphic musical notation, thus eliminating the confusion arising from teacher attempts to tell students how notes are represented. Musical symbols such as notes, rests, clef signs, etc., can be physically explored.

Tuning Peg Alteration--Violin

An interesting suggestion for altering violin tuning mechanisms is provided by Isaacs (1945): "When possible, pupils should be induced to have violin pegs bored rationally, that is to say, either at right angles or parallel to the grip" (p. 30). Students using this modified violin may change strings themselves without teacher assistance. Pegs become accessible because of students' tactile sensitivity, and problems with inserting strings into the peg box are eliminated. Besides providing another means of personal accomplishment for visually impaired musicians, this mechanical modification eliminates loss of practice time that can result while an instrument is being repaired.

Varga Violin Guide

The late Ruben Varga, a professor at the Lighthouse School in New York City, developed an important mechanical device for visually impaired violin students. Two metal rails are curved to fit over strings and parallel to the bridge, confining the bow to a specified area and preventing it from sliding forward toward the peg box.

This guide is extremely helpful, especially to beginning string players who have not yet developed level bowing. It is also helpful for more advanced students with bad habits in bowing patterns. Within a short period of time, players can acquire an adequate bowing pattern without constant help from a teacher.

Trombone Position Guide

DiPasquale (1956, p. 22) reports on a device that can be used in learning trombone positions. Since the trombone slide has no fixed marking, initial accuracy may be improved by attaching a thin plastic bar parallel to the slide. This device extends the entire length of the slide with small indentations marking each position. The bar does not interfere with slide movement, and beginning players can use it as a guide for locating positions. A device of this nature is of practical use as an aid only for beginning students. As players become more advanced, this device should be replaced by a combination of sense of touch and ear discrimination.

Adjustable Piano Rack

Students with limited sight who can read large-print music find this device important. Designed and marketed by American Printing House, the piano rack fits over upright pianos and is adjustable in terms of height and distance. A person reading large print can move the rack to a comfortable reading position without sacrificing correct body position on the piano bench.

Recorded Aid for Braille Music

In 1957, Michigan State University received a grant from the U.S. Office of Education to finance development of materials for instruction of visually impaired students in instrumental music. The Aid consists essentially of instrumental music of moderate difficulty, professionally recorded in three different styles: (a) reduced tempo without accompaniment, (b) recommended tempo without accompaniment, and (c) recommended tempo with accompaniment. Levine (1968) describes these materials as follows:

> Each set of materials consists of a tape recording in a specially designed folder, along with the brailled transcription, a large print copy (for students with low acuity), and the publisher's print edition. Any of these parts can be removed from the folder for use and then returned to the unit for storage. Labelling in both braille and ink-print is used throughout for easy identification. (p. 1)

Instrumentation includes the most commonly found musical instruments: clarinet, flute, alto saxophone, cornet, and trombone.

Each one of the three performance styles mentioned fulfills a certain teaching purpose. The reduced tempo without accompaniment allows students to follow the brailled transcription, symbol by symbol, and is paced by an audible metronome beat. Pauses at

143

phrase ends and easy reading of the entire braille score permit clarification of important interpretation aspects such as dynamics.

The segment at recommended tempo without accompaniment, provides an opportunity for listening to the entire piece as a musical entity. The music selection is presented as it should sound from beginning to end, with no exaggerated breaks.

A third version includes the solo at recommended tempo with piano accompaniment. Students can locate piano cues and interludes and develop them into proper rhythmic perspective for the entire composition.

Technology and the Future

Modern technology, including electronics and the computer, has significantly altered production of materials within the last decade. Computer transcription of braille, new methods of large print reproduction, and digital displays via magnetic recording tape are only a start. Within the next few years, improvements of present electronic equipment and new inventions should make braille and large print increasingly more available, and cumbersome braille volumes obsolete. The explanation of several technological advances illustrate how these changes will come about.

Micrographics

Microform and microfiche are means already known for the storage of large amounts of printed material within a small space. These aids can be put to use in making large-print music and literary print available to visually impaired individuals. Originally studied by the American Printing House, micrographics were later discarded because special filming was a problem for the efficient use of the system. Reproduction techniques were also not sophisticated enough. Today, however, the movement for micrographic development is again underway and supported by federal funding.

Micrographics may eventually replace the bulky braille scores currently used. A single card that is conveniently stored and does not wear out easily will become the new tool. One of the advantages of micrographics is the availability of negative or positive contrast. While positive contrast (black letters on white background) is used by many visually impaired individuals, negative image (white letters on black background) is valuable for use with students of limited vision becuase of the greater intensity afforded.

Electronic Visual Aid (EVA)

The Electronic Visual Aid is a television-type device that can be used to enlarge printed matter. Connor (1978) describes the device as follows:

A more esoteric device that is becoming fairly common in schools is the EVA, electronic visual aid. The EVA is a closed-circuit television system that magnifies up to 60 times the original size and is used by tracking the camera over the printed page and looking at an ordinary TV monitor. (p. 349)

Video tape recorders and home-use versions such as the Beta-Max can also function in providing and storing large-print music on tape. Materials may be prerecorded by others or by the visually impaired person, used, and then erased. A new device still to be marketed, the "telechord," is played in the manner of a conventional record player.

The telechord, which uses low-cost discs, presents many possibilities for visually impaired musicians. Large-print scores can be recorded and, since picture sequence speed can be varied, practice at slower rates is possible. The recorder may be adapted to include a foot switch that will advance the disc to subsequent segments.

Cassette

The cassette recorder gives visually impaired persons an inexpensive and convenient form of communication. Lowenfeld (1975) says: "Availability and ease of production should eventually allow cassettes to replace talking books previously recorded at 16 2/3 rpm and 8 1/3 rpm" (p. 187).

Two technological developments in cassette recording are particularly important to the visually impaired: speech compression and tactile display.

Speech compression

Reading speed has always been a problem in making recordings. Although the human mind can comprehend a high rate of speed, methods of production were previously unavailable. Fortunately, technology has provided the means to increase reading rates recorded on cassette machines. Lowenfeld (1975) explains:

Time compression can be achieved by increasing the playback speed. This results in what is known as the Donald Duck

145

effect by which the voice pitch becomes higher and squeaky and rather unpleasant to many listeners though it may still be understandable. There are now some methods by which speech can be compressed by discarding parts of a message within or between words so that the message is shortened without suffering in its understandability. This is done by a device called the harmonic compressor developed jointly by engineers of the Bell Laboratories and the American Foundation for the Blind. It is now possible to compress speech without the Donald Duck effect. Thus, the rate of reading can be doubled without voice distortion. (pp. 187-188)

With these new improvements, comprehension rates may be increased. Speeds of around 275 words per minute are possible and approach visual reading rates for the sighted.

Braille display

There are now available cassette recorders that will produce a tactile display of braille characters. These machines will provide an important aid to visually impaired musicians. Not only can prerecorded tapes be obtained, but visually impaired persons can record braille music characters for future use.

The capacity of these units is surprising; one ninety-minute cassette can accommodate six braille volumes. The recorder is described by Townsend (1977) as follows:

The keyboard mounted on the face of the recorder has ten keys. There are the usual keys for each dot in the braille cell, plus one key for spacing. One key permits backspacing one character at a time to correct errors. The other two keys control the blocks of 120 characters in which the data are stored before transfer to the tape. One key returns to the beginning of a 120-character block, the other transfers one 120-block to the tape, a process taking 2-3 seconds. In the latest model, just being introduced, there is no delay in transfer time from the memory to the tape, and the operator can write without stopping and without having to concern himself about the break between successive blocks of 120 cells.

When reading from a prerecorded cassette, the output is displayed on a reading board of 12 braille cells that are the same size as those used in braille books. The reader runs his or her fingers along the line of 12 characters from left to right. Upon reaching the last character, touching a switch immediately calls up the next 12 characters. In this way, the whole tape can be read, without interruption, at the reader's own speed. (p. 324)

A significant problem with this device is the current cost. French-manufactured recorders sell for about $2,500 and American ones retail from about $3,500. If these devices follow the path of calculators and early models of cassette machines, prices should eventually go down.

Computer

Computers have provided an important breakthrough in the production of braille music. The computer can transcribe in seconds what normally would take hours for a person with many years of extensive training to accomplish. More importantly, computers enable the instant mass production of materials at a greatly reduced cost. The computer at Baruch College prints braille at a rate of 120 characters per second. Any literary or music composition developed into a computer program can be printed out in braille by means of crossover networks.

Computers connected to speech synthesizers can automatically turn printed matter into electronically simulated speech. The importance of this device is paramount. By using these devices, the arduous job of transforming written prose into talking books can be simplified. Services of readers who normally spend hours at this task can be put to use elsewhere.

The music educator will be able to have texts for history, appreciation, and theory converted quickly to audio format, thereby greatly increasing instructional efficiency. At present, these devices are still at the experimental stage.

Conclusion

This paper has shown that the number of visually impaired in sighted educational programs has increased over the years, and music teachers may need to have an understanding of instructional methods and materials for effective teaching. "Mainstreaming" and redefined roles of residential schools may be considered factors that have influenced these changes.

Material needs are beginning to be met by an increasing number of technological advances. Computers can solve the need for more braille music. Large-print music is now being produced in greater quantity.

The outlook for visually impaired musicians is bright. Music educators must become aware of instructional methods and materials. Through their utilization, visually impaired musicians will be more easily accommodated into sighted music classrooms.

REFERENCES

Atkins, G., & McCarthy, G. (1962). *The electronic baton.* Unpublished paper, Perkins School for the Blind, Boston, Massachusetts.

Christie, J. (1779). Description of the theograph. *Monthly Magazine, 4,* 368-369.

Cirella, A. (1950). *Educational and vocational problems for the blind in music.* Unpublished master's thesis, New England Conservatory of Music, Boston, Massachusetts.

Coates, E. R. (1976). Music for the blind and physically handicapped from the library of congress. *American Music Teacher, 26,* 21-24.

Connor, A. (1978). Building bridges for the visually handicapped through micrographics. *Journal of Micrographics, 11,* 3-5.

Darling, L. C. (1965, October 14). Music for the blind. *Boston Sunday Herald Magazine,* 6-8.

DiPasquale, H. J. (1956). *Teaching instrumental music to the blind.* Unpublished master's thesis, Duquesne University, Pittsburgh, Pennsylvania.

Freedman, S. (1975). Psychosocial evaluation. In S. J. Spungin (Ed.), *Precollege programs for blind and visually handicapped students,* pp. 1-24. New York: American Foundation for the Blind.

Gagnepain, J. T. (1971). Music education and the blind. *Missouri Journal of Research in Music Education, 11,* 39-66.

Hoy, S. A. (1954). *The development of an adequate teaching procedure for the teaching of piano for the visually handicapped.* Unpublished master's thesis, University of South Dakota, Vermillion.

Issacs, E. (1945). *Handbook for blind teachers of music* (Vols. 1-2 of 4). London: National Institute for the Blind.

Kersten, F. (1970). Catalog of music publications. Louisville, Kentucky: American Printing House for the Blind.

Kersten, F. (1974). American printing house for the blind. In *The world book encyclopedia* (Vol. 1 of 22). Chicago, Illinois: Field Enterprises Education Corporation.

Kersten, F. (1978a). *Music catalog*. Chicago, Illinois: Johanna Bureau for the Blind and Visually Handicapped.

Kersten, F. (1978b). *The musical mainstream*. Washington, D.C.: Library of Congress, Division for the Blind.

Kersten, F. (1978c). *The braille book bank*. Rochester, New York: National Braille Association.

Kersten, F. (1979). *Music programs at residential schools for the blind*. Unpublished research study.

Kircher, B. J. (1979). *The visually handicapped student: College music degree programs*. Unpublished master's thesis, State University of New York, Potsdam.

Levine, S. J. (1968). *A recorded aid for braille* (Tape recording). East Lansing, Michigan: Michigan State University Regional Instructional Materials Center for Handicapped Children and Youth.

Lowenfeld, B. (1975). Psychological problems of children with impaired vision. In W. M. Cruickshank (Ed.), *Psychology of exceptional children and youth* (4th ed.) (pp. 100-135). Englewood Cliffs, New Jersey: Prentice-Hall.

McCarthy, G. (1958). *Vocational guidance for professional music*. Unpublished manuscript. Perkins School for the Blind, Boston, Massachusetts.

Patrick, P. H. (1976). *Computer-printing of braille music using the I.M.L.- M.I.R. system documentation*. Unpublished manuscript. American University, Washington, D.C.

Reuss, A. (1935). Development and problems of musical notation for the blind. New York: New York Institute.

Townsend, A. H. (1977). Sensory aids ELINFA portable braille cassette recorder. *Journal of Visual Impairment and Blindness, 71*, 324.

PLAYING INSTRUMENTS WITH THE BLIND AND SEVERELY VISUALLY HANDICAPPED

by

HELMUT MOOG

It is understandable that music plays an important role in the lives of the blind and severely visually handicapped. Persons who are denied the aesthetic experience of the visual world should have every opportunity to be exposed to those aesthetic areas that are accessible without eyesight, most especially poetry and music.[1] It will always be difficult for the blind to gain complete access to the fine arts. Investigating sculptures by feeling, for example, is only possible with certain size sculptures. Valuable pieces, moreover, are cautiously set up out of reach in museums so that, as with paintings and drawings, mediating explanations and interpretations of sighted persons are necessary.

Since the blind are trained in music in general through their remaining auditory capacity, the loss of visual information (and, because of this, an increased importance in auditory information) leads to a corresponding necessity for music education. The blind and severely visually handicapped need music education for yet another reason: music education not only develops listening skills for musical elements and themes but also for all kinds of auditory information. Transfer effects derived from the auditory training through music are of special value to the blind. By transfer effects we mean that exercises in one area lead to more achievement in another area. Some of the most significant transfer effects of music are the emotional, intellectual, and social benefits that are provided.

Music is accessible to the blind through a non-handicapped sense. However, the widespread notion that every blind person is unusually musically gifted needs some clarification. Blindness is not something that strikes only the highly musically gifted.[2] It is much more likely that inborn musicality--whose relationship to musicality

---

[1]F. Goodenough and D. Goodenough, "The Importance of Music in the Life of a Visually Handicapped Child," in *The Education of the Visually Handicapped,* ed. Association for Education of the Visually Handicapped (Philadelphia, Pennsylvania: Association for Education of the Visually Handicapped, 1970), pp. 28-32.

[2]Derek J. Pitman, "The Musical Ability of Blind Children," *Research Bulletin of the American Foundation of the Blind* 11 (1965):63.

induced by training is still unknown--is distributed among the blind in the same way as among sighted persons.[3] It is more probable that the remaining senses, including hearing, are more highly developed because of the demands placed on them.[4] Empirical investigations have ascertained that, especially in auditory perception tests and musical memory achievement tests, blind persons score higher than sighted ones.[5]

Nevertheless, we must clarify another conception about the musical ability of the blind. In more advanced cultures, access to music paradoxically happens to a great extent through visual information. The blind, however, cannot use notation either for practice or performance purposes. When they are playing in an orchestra or other ensemble, they can not receive cues from the conductor. Plastic notes and Braille notes have limited usefulness since they can be used during music making only with those instruments that require one hand.[6] These tactile tools are useful only in developing musical concepts. However, the performance itself must be carried out by heart. Another problem with these notes is that they give information at the same time as the music comes into existence. Therefore, these plastic and Braille notes lack an important advantage of visual notes, that is, allowing to a certain extent a simultaneous overview of the succession of tones.

A sighted instrumental student is able to look at finger movements when the teacher demonstrates certain passages, and he is able to imitate it and may control his own motoric achievements visually. His music may be marked to show where an exercise or a repetition begins, and fingering and other markings can be written down. The blind student is denied all of these aids. It is

---

[3]E. E. Seashore and T. L. Ling, "The Comparative Sensitiveness of Blind and Seeing Persons," *Psychological Monographs* 25 (1918):148-58.

[4]M. Neuhaeuser, "Das Orff-Schulwerk in der Blindenschule," *Der Blindenfreund* 76 (1956):119.

[5]J. Kwalwasser, *Exploring the Musical Mind*, p. 108 (New York: Colman Ross, 1955); Pitman, pp. 64-69; R. M. Drake, "Factorial Analysis of Music by Spearman Tetrad Difference Technique," *Journal of Musicology* 1 (1939):7-10.

[6]M. Neuhaeuser, "Musikerziehung bei Blinden," in *Mit den Händen sehen. 125 Jahre Blindenanstalt Dueren*, ed. Landschaftsverband Rheinland (Duesseldorf: Landschaftsverband Rheinland, 1970):39-47.

particularly difficult for the blind student learning a string instrument, because it appears that visual control is a greater factor in mastering all the different positions governed by the bow and the instrument during music making. It is logical that a blind person has special obstacles to overcome when learning a string instrument.

The blind experience an unusual paradox concerning music. On the one hand, there is a need to receive music education, far above that of any other group of handicapped people; on the other hand, blind persons have to overcome these special obstacles in learning music.

Before World War I, the reasons for special music education had been identified. For the blind, there were two innovations that opened up two new roads: the development of music notation for the blind, in which tactile Braille notes are used; and the introduction of piano and organ lessons in schools for the blind.

Braille notation allows the blind person to examine music without the assistance of others. He touches the notation with one hand and plays the notes he has "read" with the other. Of course, he can also sing the music he has read. However, as every musician knows, it is far more difficult to sing at sight than to play at sight. This difference in difficulty lies in the fact that sightreading instrumental music implies a direct relationship between a note and a grip on the instrument being used. This first sightreading is possible without having any concept of the melody being played. Sightsinging a melody, on the other hand, is more difficult because one cannot anticipate the concept of the melody.

The second innovation prior to World War I in music education for the blind was the introduction of piano and organ lessons in schools for the blind. Today, this particular selection of instruments seems rather one-sided. However, considering the historical context, the innovation seems more valid. The reason for giving piano and organ lessons was the profound need of the blind for music education. At the time--before the beginning of the era of mass media--the piano repertoire was not limited to works written specifically for that instrument but included arrangements of orchestral compositions as well. The piano can make it possible for a blind person to have a more varied approach to music literature. Before keyboard instruments were used, this goal could be achieved only by using notation. For this reason, Braille notation was created. Even though the blind person cannot play the piano with both hands and touch the notation at the same time, he is still in a position to read a piece of music without the help of others. The combination of Braille notation and the piano is also a sensible one since making music with one hand and touching notation with the other is really possible only with keyboard instruments.

As early as the beginning of this century, applications were delivered to authorities by educators of the blind to buy large numbers of pianos. These authorities complied with that request--a credit to both the educators and administrators for their insight. Some schools for the blind still require piano lessons.

We know that piano and organ lessons in schools for the blind were successful. An impressive example of this success is the internationally known blind organist, Helmut Wahcha. However, in spite of the number of successful students, there are still many--too many--whose success is not commensurate with the amount of diligent practicing they have devoted to the instrument. In addition, the problems of ensemble playing have not been solved, but avoided, and the loneliness of the blind continues to grow because of the limitations of keyboard instruments.

Much has changed during the last decades. There have been strides made in ensemble playing for the blind musician. After first using keyboard instruments, then wind and percussion instruments, the guitar and mandolin have now been introduced into music education programs for the blind.[7] Wind instruments, percussion instruments, and some plucked instruments are easier to play well in a short time than keyboard instruments. They are also easier to play in an ensemble. It seems that longer lessons and more diligent, successful practicing with plucked and wind instruments will bring the blind student more gratification and achievement. There is much ensemble literature for wind and plucked instruments that is useful with players who have only been playing a short while. These instruments can allow blind children the opportunity to make music with sighted players as well as with other blind musicians.

Those instruments that are played with hand positions remaining in more or less the same place and for which motoric skill is limited to the fingers are the most advantageous for blind persons. For this reason, woodwind, brass, and wind instruments are the best choice. Finger dexterity and tone production by means of correct breathing can be learned without visual aids.

Blind players often have difficulty taking apart or reassembling their instruments. The problems of notation, however, have been somewhat solved. Acoustic technical media have begun a

---

[7]Neuhaeuser, p. 124.

new chapter in the music education of the blind. Prior to this, blind instrumental students learned only from Braille notation. Now, however, beginners can dispense with this notation system; tape recordings of pieces and instrumental exercises are better learning tools.

Since one of the aims in music education for the blind is to help students learn to hear, why then should blind players not learn by hearing? This means that all exercises and short pieces must be taped before blind instrumental students can learn to play by hearing. As it stands, they must learn to play by heart anyway. Experience with this method has shown that the blind learn more easily and faster and, at the same time, get an idea of the interpretation of the piece being learned.[8] Without this audiotape, the teacher is the only guide to leading the students from merely playing notes to making music. Through listening to the tape, however, the student can discover the piece on his own--its expressive qualities, melodic and formal structures, the important themes. Last but not least, a teacher can explain a point more easily with auditory examples than with a tactile notation system. Therefore, Braille notation is no longer necessary to teach beginning blind students to play wind or plucked instruments.

Those blind students, however, who intend to go on in music, to become professional musicians or scholars, must learn Braille notation. They must be encouraged to do so to the point that they can sightread fluently. The so-called "Music Minus One" records are of great value to the blind musician. These recordings have both solo part and accompaniment recorded together on one side, and the accompaniment alone on the other side. The solo part is to be played by the student. It would be better still to have a third recording in which the solo part was provided by itself.

Making music with instruments is only part of musical reality, and also of music education. The different goals of sightreading on an instrument or vocally make it obvious that a combination of vocal and instrumental playing is desirable. Moreover, movement response to music is part of a well-balanced program. The advent and use of Braille notation and keyboard lessons into schools for the blind was a limited idea to begin with. Let us not limit ourselves in the programs that we now create for the blind.

---

[8]Wilhelm Heinrichs, "Zum Einsatz von Blasinstrumenten bei Blinden und hochgradig Sehbehinderten," in *Blasinstrumente bei Behinderten,* ed. Helmut Moog. (Tutzing: Schneider, 1978), p. 121.

REFERENCES

Drake, R. M. "Factorial Analysis of Music by Spearman Tetrad Difference Technique." *Journal of Musicology* 1 (1939):6-10.

Goodenough, F., and Goodenough, D. "The Importance of Music in the Life of a Visually Handicapped Child." In *The Education of the Visually Handicapped*, pp. 28-32. Edited by the Association for the Education of the Visually Impaired. Philadelphia, Pennsylvania: Association for the Education of the Visually Impaired, 1970.

Heinrichs, Wilhelm. "Zum Einsatz von Blasinstrumenten bei Blinden und hochgradig Sehbehinderten." In *Blasinstrumente bei Behinderten*, pp. 117-26. Edited by Helmut Moog. Tutzing: Schneider, 1978.

Kwalwasser, J. *Exploring the Musical Mind*. New York: Colman Ross, 1955.

Moog, Helmut. "Zur Situation der Musik in den Blinden- und Sehbehindertenschulen der Bundesrepublik." *Zeitschrift für das Blinden- und Sehbehindertenbildungswesen (Der Blindenfreund)* 97 (1977):84-89.

Neuhaeuser, M. "Das Orff-Schulwerk in der Blindenschule." Der Blindenfreund 76 (1956):116-31.

_____. "Lebensnahe Musikerziehung." *Der Blindenfreund* 82 (1962):153-65.

_____. "Musikerziehung bei Blinden." *Mit den Händen sehen. 125 Jahre Blindenanstalt Dueren*, pp. 39-47. Edited by Landschaftsverband Rheinland, 1970. Duesseldorf: Landschaftsverband Rheinland, 1970.

Pitman, Derek J. "The Musical Ability of Blind Children." *Research Bulletin of the American Foundation of the Blind* 11 (1965):63-79.

Seashore, E. E., and Ling, T. L. "The Comparative Sensitiveness of Blind and Seeing Persons." *Psychological Monographs* 25 (1918): 148-58.

REPORT ON A PROJECT WITH AUTISTIC
CHILDREN AT INDIANA UNIVERSITY

by

ALICE JACOBS

Among many other duties, the school special music teacher is occasionally included as a member of a team of professionals who follow the progress of each individual child. Before the end of each school year, a parent-teacher conference is held to discuss the individual educational programming for each child. The parents, school principal, regular and special classroom teachers, school psychologist, and others participate in this formal conference to establish long- and short-term objectives and annual educational goals. The development of the I.E.P. (Individualized Education Program) is based upon frequent assessments of work, progress, medical reports, teacher observations and evaluations, and other pertinent information.

The music teacher is often called upon to submit data and advice at these conferences. Training for these meetings and other special duties usually occurs through inservice workshops held by the school. Observations of the child should be recorded, the student's work discussed, and any helpful suggestions or changes noted on daily reports or logs that frequently are requested at such I.E.P. conferences. As P. L. 94-142 mandates, there shall be an annual review of records, careful observations, and recorded data for each special education child enrolled in school.

These duties are the legal obligations of every public, private, or residential educational facility and its personnel. The institution must also require its personnel to recommend, understand, and defend any pupil assessment, diagnosis, or placement. The music teacher is no less responsible than any other professional involved in the case conferences, assessment procedures, or educational planning made in the name of the most appropriate situation for any handicapped child. Music educators must understand the concept of prescriptive teaching, which signifies that as the school year progresses, a curriculum should be devised and amended based on observational and measurable data. The special music teacher would need to be able to recognize deficient learning skills and plan activities specifically designed to remediate these deficits and, at the same time, continue to teach musical skills and concepts. These responsibilities demand that such teachers, in addition to being musicians, teachers, and specialists of learning problems, should also have sufficient educational background and expertise.

157

The emotionally disturbed child, who is the most frequent candidate for regular class placement (or, at least, partial regular class placement), is most likely to be in contact with every educator in a public school at one time or another. Due to the increase in social pressures, divorce, one-parent families, and financial strains of daily living, emotional disturbance in youngsters can be expected to escalate. The emotionally disturbed student might be academically up to par with other peers of his age group; on the other hand, he might also be below level in one or many areas. Remedial instruction might therefore be required. Music, however, is one class where these children are commonly found on a regular class status.

As with all other exceptionalities, emotional disturbance may range in severity from mild and moderate to severe and profound. During class time, mildly handicapped students might have occasional outbursts that could be handled with a strong verbal reprimand from the teacher, or a few minutes in a time-out room. Otherwise, the child, along with others, might attend an informal therapy session directed by school personnel such as a psychologist or a team of qualified teachers. If the child's condition is severe, it is quite possible that facilities would be difficult to find and that he or she might therefore be sent to an assessment center for extensive testing, experimental curriculum development, or special placement considerations on a residential basis.

Based upon the recommendations of the regular school teachers, principal, parents, and other professional personnel, e.g., social worker, school psychologist, mental health clinic advisor, etc., a child may be sent to an assessment center such as the Developmental Training Center in Bloomington, Indiana. Upon entry to the center, the child undergoes individual psychological and educational testing, a medical examination, and an interview with both the child and parents. In addition, some children are seen by a psychiatrist if such a request is made by the psychologist, teacher, or parent. Such a request is made if there is a possibility of neurological impairment or psychoses. The parents are also interviewed by the center staff to collect data pertaining to the child's history.

A major concern of many educators is often the question of establishing control with autistic children. For the behaviorists and developmental therapists, the key is to have a highly structured environment. Oppenheim (1977) recommends several crucial steps in working with these difficult students:

1. Contain the child in the teaching situation. Explain that completion of the task is dependent upon remaining in the chair until it is time to do something else.

2. A teacher or other instructor must follow up throughout all commands given to the student. At no time should avoidance of a task be permitted due to a tantrum, aggression, or other negative behavior. If there is evidence of an inability to complete the task or an unwillingness to comply, take the child's hands and literally put him through the physical motions of the task. Ignore any complaints that the child makes about this technique and remind him or her that you "had to help him because he did not follow directions on his own." The child will usually ask to be given another chance to complete the task on his own in order to save his pride.

3. Limit the duration of the task. Special children, in general, are unable to attend to tasks that are complicated or lengthy in nature. They become impatient, frustrated, or easily distracted. Symptoms of their need to change the task include: fidgeting, humming, hitting, kicking, or daydreaming. These children may eventually be trained to verbalize their need to do something different once the original task has been completed. A gradual increase in the task and reinforcement times must be carefully planned. The child should not be expected to remain in his seat for more than twenty minutes. An equal amount of free time is needed in order to demonstrate that successful completion of an assignment will not go unnoticed or unrewarded. This, in turn, will breed the desire to have similar experiences.

4. At the outset of a teaching program with an autistic child, and for some time after, instruction should occur on a one-to-one basis. One cannot overemphasize the fact that autistic children will all too eagerly withdraw from a situation or become aggressive and/or violent rather than be in contact with other people. There must first be the development of comfort and trust with just one other person before the child can become involved in a small group. Regardless of the physical environment, control must be established from the start of any session, and it must be discussed again at the beginning of each subsequent meeting.

For each meeting with a child, the writer often carries along a chart of procedures and expected behaviors that is read either by the child or the writer. Such a chart proves to be a very effective reminder as it creates security, structure, and control for the children involved. Autistic children need this structure from external sources since they are incapable of imposing such discipline by themselves. They will attempt to test one's rules and

159

regulations quite often since every new situation is threatening to their isolationism. It is at that point that one must quietly remind them of the procedure chart that was read together before the start of the lesson. This technique is equally effective with group instruction, although the focus of restrictions might need to change. Instead of reinforcing a single behavior, an entire array of behaviors must be specifically outlined on the chart so that every child's requirements for order have been mentioned. Control should never become synonymous with irrational, dictatorial power that stifles any individuality of response that the child might attempt.

Materials used with autistic students should be individualized as much as possible. Rarely do they all possess similar interests, ability levels, or musical capabilities. Some are advanced socially while others are more intellectually superior. Some may lack adequate fine-motor control and are not yet capable of working with musical instruments such as the recorder or piano. Many different combinations of skills can and do exist within one classroom of autistic children. An emphasis on individual instruction would lessen the opportunity for failure, disinterest, withdrawal, or aggression that often arises when these children are expected to perform together for an entire period. Certain individual activities may complement successful participation in group work.

As Alvin (1975) explains:

Music can contribute to the general growth of the handicapped child in many ways: as a substitute for other activities; as a compensation since it can bring reward and achievement; as an agent of sensory development; as an emotional outlet; as a mental stimulus; as a means of socialization. These many aspects of a single factor give music an integrating power because they are indissolubly linked with one another and they involve the mind, body, and emotion of the child in one experience.

In teaching music, especially to the handicapped population, one must never lose sight of the fact that music need not be just an end in itself. The ultimate goal should be that the child makes a healthy and satisfactory adjustment to his/her environment and that this adjustment should be aided through acceptable behavior, creativity, and expressive communication, using music as one possible medium.

The four autistic subjects used in this study resided for five days a week at the Developmental Training Center in Bloomington, Indiana. Residence at this assessment center is for only one year. As a member of the recreational therapy department with no previous experience in teaching music to severely disturbed children, the writer's first step was to observe them in order to assess their musical skills. After approximately one month of observation, the students' patterns of behavior, motivational needs, physical coordination, fine- and gross-motor skills, language capabilities, and musical interests were carefully recorded. Since the only musical experience offered was during group activities, plans were originally made to maintain this format in order that the children would be accustomed to seeing the writer and begin to trust her before beginning individual music sessions. Though there were six students residing at the center, only four were chosen as subjects. The other two were extremely aggressive and showed no musical interests or abilities.

The musical activities included both group sessions and private, individualized lessons on an instrument prescribed for each child. A thorough study of personal records, including mental and family histories, plus suggestions from other members of the staff, were taken into account prior to making assignments for private lessons. It became necessary during the course of the preliminary investigations to modify an original decision: a different instrument was recommended for one of the subjects since her interests and the strength of reinforcers began to develop in different directions than was initially intended. Group sessions were conducted by the recreational therapist with the assistance of the writer. Included in each child's curriculum were: (a) two assessments--initial and revised, (b) two I.E.P. objectives--pre- and postinstructional, (c) individual lesson summaries, and (d) "can do" and "next step" recommendations--present and future levels of performance competencies based upon the task analysis format.

Practice time was arranged with the home programmers who reside at the assessment center with these children. The length and frequency of practice varied from child to child and from day to day. As these students attended classes from 8:30 A.M. to 5:00 P.M. each day, there were many other assignments given to them by their regular subject teachers. Insistence upon regular practice time was not possible under these circumstances.

The length of each individual lesson was set at approximately 10-15 minutes, as their attention spans and concentration levels could not tolerate much more. At times, however, lessons were curtailed for emotional, physical, or other reasons. Discussing the underlying problems that might cause the child to become extremely abusive or aggressive became much more important than trying to maintain attention on music.

The location of the lessons was another crucial consideration in planning musical activities. Autistic children need a rigid routine in order to maximize their level of concentration and understanding, while minimizing emotional outbursts and/or tantrums that might be caused by the most subtle environmental change. They are keenly aware of all noises, sound, or disturbances that are extraneous to the task. One boy felt comfortable having his lessons in his bedroom at the center. Eventually he was encouraged to come down to the living room where another boy was quietly working. This flexibility avoided any confrontations and allowed the student to feel secure enough to attend to music lessons. For this young boy who was particularly sensitive to sounds and people who entered into his isolated "physical space," moving to a more open, possibly threatening situation was a remarkable improvement. The next part of the paper is a brief description of the boy's musical instruction and progress.

Randy (age 11)

Based upon personal observations during group music, Randy seemed to show interest in most musical activities. His attention span was short, however, and he often needed several distractions or cues, and/or possibly even some demonstrations of appropriate behavior during music. He seemed to get along well with peers except when they came too close to him. He became involved in music activities as long as he was spoken to directly and when he was given a specific, direct task that required a specified number of repetitions. If the rules and expectations of behavior were spelled out specifically prior to the beginning of the session, Randy was usually able to follow the entire lesson to its end.

When Randy was asked to sing a song or recite the words to a new melody, he became extremely compliant, eager to please everyone and extremely attentive to any musical activities. He was able to carry a tune, match pitch, and had a remarkable memory for both melodies and verses. In addition, he had a sense of beat that he clearly exhibited when listening to a record. He usually clapped his hands or beat a drum in exact time unless the tempo became too slow for him to pay strict attention. It was decided that Randy should learn to play the recorder since he had excellent muscular coordination and needed immediate success with a musical instrument. It was felt that learning the piano would require attention and patience beyond his capabilities. By the end of the twelfth individual lesson on the recorder, certain information came to light:

1. Randy would begin to daydream when he was feeling "overloaded" by new information or when he could no longer attend to the task at hand.

2. He needed to have names for each of his fingers in order to differentiate between them (e.g., "Mr. Thumb and Mr. Index").

3. All instruction had to be imitative in nature since he could not retain verbal information and be expected to translate it into physical movement, no matter how simple the instructions were.

4. The best strategy that worked with Randy was to give him the *exact* number of times he must correctly perform a task.

5. Full and constant eye contact had to be maintained in order to ensure that Randy would perform the task at all. If not, he would either begin to daydream or become extremely frustrated to the point of throwing a tantrum.

Final recommendations for Randy included:

1. Randy's imitative rhythmic skills should be utilized by transferring them to exercises on drums, bells, or other rhythm instruments. It was too much to ask him to incorporate the rhythm, notes, and fingerings required on the recorder. While initial success was attained, progress was not consistent beyond a certain point of difficulty.

2. There should be a gradual increase in the length of rhythmic patterns to be imitated.

3. Imitation of melodies should be gradually introduced. These tunes should be sung without words and then transferred to musical notation in order to begin the process of music reading.

4. At this point, the recorder should be re-introduced, incorporating Randy's new rhythmic and music reading abilities.

5. Randy's attention span should be lengthened by increasing the number of patterns or melodies he must imitate within any given period of time. Songs that Randy knows and sings are highly motivating to him and work best to maintain his attention.

6. Music is a source of much joy to Randy. He enjoyed the individual attention given to him during the lessons as well as the group approval of his short performances on the recorder. However, it was expecting too much of him to ask him to incorporate several skills at once. He was eager to learn, to please others, and to

enjoy musical activities of all types. Therefore, to refuse him the opportunity to resume individualized instruction because of his behavioral setback would be a terrible injustice.

Autistic children who initially appeared to be so withdrawn or aggressive were transformed into more normalized students each time they had individual music lessons. They thrived on the personal attention and verbal praise given to them during private periods away from everyone else. They began to internalize these good feelings and look forward to making more progress on their instrument. Though one girl developed arthritis, and another boy regressed to a more rudimentary level, all four students involved in this study continued to show interest in music in spite of these setbacks.

Imagine, however, if music had *not* been a part of their curriculum. How else would they have expressed their individuality? They certainly could not have done so in math, reading, or gym. Music reached out to these children without requiring any previous musical skills. They had never played a recorder or autoharp before, nor had they been asked to imitate rhythmic patterns. This lack of exposure to music is due to the fact that these children were never before offered the opportunity to participate in musical activities to the extent that they had been during the year they lived at the residential center in Bloomington, Indiana.

Since not all the subjects of this project were to become budding musical geniuses, the writer strove to attain a compromise between being a performance-oriented educator and a scientific-minded therapist. Instead, these students were approached by a teacher who had a determined, positive, and inquisitive attitude; who set reasonable and attainable goals; who received excellent instructional support; and who created the necessary structure and control to enable these students to function at their own levels. These attributes were coupled with a developmental behavioral plan that assumed that assets were to be emphasized, while deficits were to be paid as little regard as possible.

It was hoped that the resulting contacts with music would be some of the most rewarding, successful, and enlightening experiences of these children's lives. This project added a new dimension to this researcher's musical life, one that had never before been considered nor explored in any music course offered by a university.

THE THEORETICAL BASIS FOR THE USE OF MUSIC THERAPY WITH APHASIC PATIENTS

by

DALE B. TAYLOR

Aphasia is a disturbance of language resulting from damage to the brain. The brain uses language symbols for speaking, reading, writing, and listening. Comprehension of speech entering through the auditory tract requires use of Wernicke's area. Damage to either Wernicke's area or Broca's area would result in impaired speaking ability. The visual cortex, angular gyrus, and Wernicke's area are necessary for reading. Wernicke's area, angular gyrus, visual cortex, and Broca's area are all involved in reading aloud and in writing and are all located in the left cranial hemisphere. While the left hemisphere carries on primarily verbal and logical behaviors, the right hemisphere has been found to be more active for nonverbal, holistic functions. These include singing and most other musical skills. Because singing can be regained with left hemisphere damage, the right hemisphere, through melodic verbal activities, may be used to assist those clients having speech impairments resulting from such damage.

Although there are many forms in which the illness manifests itself, aphasia can be defined as a disturbance of language resulting from damage to the brain. There is identifiable impairment in the use of language symbols. This paper will: (a) identify the four primary uses of language symbols; (b) localize and specify the functions of the four cranial areas involved in the manipulation of language symbols; (c) cite recent findings concerning hemispheric dominance in the processing of musical behavior; and (d) propose a model based on hemispheric specializations for the use of brain portions concerned with music to assist in the rehabilitation of persons whose cranial speech areas have been damaged.

Human beings use language symbols to accomplish four primary modes of behavior: speaking, reading, writing, and listening. Although the processing and manipulation of these symbols include other behaviors such as learning, remembering, sequencing, or recalling, the primary behaviors involved in receiving or expressing language symbols are speaking, reading, writing, and listening.

Listening

When a word is heard, the output from the primary auditory area of the temporal lobe is received by Wernicke's area, which lies immediately adjacent to the primary auditory area. Damage to Wernicke's area would cause an aphasic loss of speech comprehension.

Speaking

If the word is to be spoken, the auditory pattern is transmitted via a nerve bundle known as the arcuate fasciculus from Wernicke's area to Broca's area, located adjacent to the region of the brain that controls the muscles of speech. Here the articulatory form is aroused for use by the motor area in coordinating the speech musculature. Damage to Broca's or Wernicke's area results in impairment in speaking ability.

Reading

When a word is to be read silently, the output from the primary visual cortex is sent to the angular gyrus, a region located immediately posterior to Wernicke's area. There, the visual stimulus is converted into the auditory form for use by Wernicke's area. When it is received in Wernicke's area, the auditory form of the word is transmitted to association areas for speech comprehension. If the word is to be read aloud, the pattern is sent to Broca's area for use as described above. Damage to the visual cortex, angular gyrus, or Wernicke's area will result in impaired reading ability.

Writing

If a word is to be written, auditory recall of the word is formulated in Wernicke's area, transmitted via the angular gyrus to the visual cortex to facilitate visual recall of its written form, and passed finally to Broca's area, where instructions for coordination of digital musculature are formulated and activated. Damage to any but the visual area will result in impaired writing ability.

Damage to Wernicke's area results in difficulty in comprehending both spoken and written language. One would be unable to speak, repeat, and write correctly. The fact that speech is fluent and well articulated in such cases suggests that Broca's area is intact but receiving inadequate information. If the damage were in Broca's area, the effect of the lesion would be to disrupt articulation. Speech would be slow and labored, but comprehension would remain intact.

Two important extensions of the Wernicke model were advanced by a French neurologist, Joseph Jules Dejerine. In 1891, he described a disorder called alexia with agraphia: the loss of the ability to read and write. The patient could, however, speak and understand spoken language. Postmortem examination showed that there was a lesion in the angular gyrus of the left hemisphere, the area of the brain that acts as a way station between the visual and the auditory regions. A lesion here would separate the visual and auditory language areas. Although words and letters would be seen correctly, they would be meaningless visual patterns, since the visual pattern must first be converted to the auditory form before the word can be comprehended. Conversely, the auditory pattern for a word must be transformed into the visual pattern before the word can be spelled out. Patients suffering from alexia with agraphia cannot recognize words spelled aloud to them nor can they themselves spell aloud a spoken word.

In order to use music to help the aphasic person regain these functions, the separate functions of the right and left hemispheres must be understood. While the left hemisphere carries on primarily verbal, sequential, and logical behaviors, the right hemisphere functions in a more nonverbal, holistic, spatial manner. Research has shown that although the left hemisphere appears to be used more effectively for identifying minute changes in frequency, the right hemisphere demonstrates greater accuracy for intensity discriminations.

The right hemisphere has also been found to be dominant for the perception of musical chords. In addition, it has been found to be necessary for singing. Because singing can be regained with left hemisphere impairment, it should follow that the use of the right hemisphere through singing or melodic verbal activities may assist those clients whose speaking ability is impaired by left hemisphere damage. This assistance is possible because, in the normal healthy brain, the two hemispheres communicate with each other via the corpus callosum at the rate of four billion impulses per second.

Right hemisphere dominance for melodic and harmonic perception suggests that guided listening experiences may assist the individual whose comprehension of spoken language is impaired by damage to Wernicke's area. This becomes extremely important in view of the involvement of Wernicke's area in all four of the primary uses of language symbols.

The right hemisphere is used in both auditory and visual pattern discriminations such as those necessary for reading music. Reading music and singing, or reading music and playing an instrument may therefore be a useful technique for using the right hemisphere to help regain some functions in clients suffering from an aphasic loss of reading or writing ability.

Although these proposals await an adequate pool of aphasic clients for thorough clinical testing, they are proposed here as a theoretical model for further investigation with available subjects in appropriate situations. For those who may have access to a group of aphasic clients, some specific suggestions can be made based on literature appearing during the past two decades.

1. Music therapy for the aphasic client must be tailored to each individual client in order to maximize its effectiveness in treating the specific speech and language disorders of that person.

2. Tempos must be considerably slower than normal to decrease the strain of perceiving and forming syllables rapidly.

3. The songs used should have very few words and frequent repetition of fairly regular rhythmic patterns.

4. Each song should be sung more than once in order to give clients the opportunity to correct errors.

5. Very large song cards, showing one song only, should be used. The leader should point to the words as they are sung. This will maximize output with the least amount of strain.

6. There should be separate work and attention given to gaining improvement in those components of vocal production that are common to singing and to speaking. These components include: tempo, rhythm, pitch control, loudness, timbre, comprehension, articulation, sightreading, and song writing. Success in each of these areas can generate motivation to use all available parts of the brain and thereby achieve greater success in language functioning.

REFERENCES

Eccles, J. C. (1973). *The understanding of the brain.* New York: McGraw-Hill.

Gates, A., & Bradshaw, J. L. (1977). The role of cerebral hemispheres in music. *Brain and Language, 4,* 403-431.

Geschwind, N. (1972). Language and the brain. *Scientific American, 226,* 76-83.

Hodges, D. A. (1980). *Handbook of music psychology.* Washington, DC: National Association for Music Therapy.

Kimura, D. (1961). Cerebral dominance and the perception of verbal stimuli. *Canadian Journal of Psychology, 15,* 156-165.

Klinger, H., & Peter, D. (1963). Techniques in group singing for aphasics. In E. H. Schneider (Ed.), *Music Therapy 1962* (pp. 108-112). Washington, DC: National Association for Music Therapy.

Radocy, R, & Boyle, J. D. (1979). *Psychological foundations of musical behavior.* Springfield, Illinois: C. C. Thomas.

Roederer, J. G. (1975). *Introduction to physics and psychophysics of music* (2nd ed.). New York: Springer-Verlag.

THE POWER OF MUSIC IN PRISON

by

THOMAS G. ELLIOT and CHRISTOPHER MCGAHAN

It is well known that music has a powerful effect on human beings. Musicians strive to evoke that power through refined teaching and performance. Since music has the power to move people, teachers of music have the power to influence the direction of that movement. However, music teachers must first recognize this power and then learn how to apply it.

The extraordinary implications of this premise began to unfold for the authors in 1976, when a maximum security prison in Massachussetts was shaken by a massive riot involving more than two hundred inmates. They broke out of the assembly hall after watching the movie *Dog Day Afternoon* and began setting fires in the compound and smashing windows. A group of inmates barricaded themselves in the school library and burned books. When fifty armed corrections officers surrounded the library, the men alleged grievances and demanded a meeting with the superintendent. After several hours of negotiation, the men agreed to come out and the superintendent agreed to hear their complaints. Their list of nine demands included longer visiting hours and better food. To the surprise of everyone, a music program ranked third on the list.

In response, the Governor of Massachussetts contacted officials of the University of Lowell College of Music (located within fifteen miles of the prison) and asked for help. Dr. Elliot, then Dean of the College, agreed to meet with prison officials to explore the possibilities of a music program behind the walls. What began as an attempt merely to ameliorate the prison atmosphere through music turned out to be a significant research project using music as a rehabilitative tool.

After six years of teaching and research behind the walls, the writers are convinced that music is one of the potentially most effective instruments for rehabilitation available to present-day society.

Experts in the field of criminal behavior have long argued that rehabilitation requires treatment. They further argue that treatment is a dynamic process that cannot succeed without both the cooperation and the active, voluntary participation of the offender. Furthermore, the best environment for treatment is one that replicates a healthy social and cultural milieu--a condition thus far unachievable in the prison setting.

170

Those who have taught music in the public schools know that with each school, irrespective of the socio-economic conditions from which the students come, must create a healthy social and cultural atmosphere in order to teach successfully. That such an approach would be equally essential in the prison setting was not considered by the writers at the beginning of this program.

With due recognition of the unique characteristics of both the clientele and the setting, it was concluded that the prison students and the writers' public school students were essentially the same in that both faced identical socio-psychological challenges, and both experienced doubt and anxiety in the face of uncertainty. The most salient difference between the two groups was that while one enjoyed the freedom of society and its goods, the other was physically confined and stripped of worldly possessions. The inmates' captive status, however, provided two important advantages: (1) the stability of population, location, and daily routine; and (2) the sharp definition of human behavior caused by the extreme conditions of prison environment. Observations of these behaviors led to the further conclusion that our interactions with inmate-students on a daily basis was developing on two distinct levels: the verbal, or explicit level; and the nonverbal, or implicit level.

At the verbal level, the program consisted of music theory, instrumental music, and vocal music, all of which required the voluntary, active participation of each individual. At the nonverbal level, daily interactions were directly addressing individual psychological and social needs.

The music program was developing into a vehicle that was helping a substantial number of men to focus on their needs and life circumstances in concrete terms. In concentrating on their social and psychological needs, the nonverbal level seemed to be enhancing the verbal one. That is, the explicit value of involvement in the music program was greatly enhanced and sustained by the implicit but active nonverbal interaction.

Whether or not they knew it, the inmates' decisions to participate in the music program also made possible a legitimate opportunity for them to develop a stake in conformity, an attribute normally not found in the deviant personality. In other words, these inmates were not only mastering a musical skill but were also simultaneously rebuilding their lives. Participation required the inmates to make positive decisions and then to follow up by taking concrete actions. Both are contrary to the normal expectations of that environment; and it can be extremely difficult for offenders to make positive decisions. The individual inmate's decision to

171

participate in the music program is therefore highly significant in that it demonstrated that, under proper circumstances, the inmate can mobilize the strengths needed to achieve positive social goals.

With the passage of time it became clear that, while the importance of the musical objectives did not decrease, nevertheless the importance of these interactions as therapy increased substantially. The subtle changes noted in the behavior of each participant became more important than the success or failure of each to master any given musical task. In short order, the program itself had taken on a new cast. In the beginning, seventeen individuals appeared at the music room door. These men did not necessarily know each other, nor did they care about social interaction or group protocol. Each was insistent upon individual attention and time. Later in the program, they appeared for their 9:00 A.M. lessons in groups. They immediately took their assigned seats and, with little ado, took up as a group the routine of counting and drill.

Line trading became a favorite device for counting and playing in time. All of the men kept the beat while the melody was passed from one to another in the framework of the uniform count. When one missed a beat, the others would "jump on his case;" and when all members were successful, they would cheer themselves as a group. Through techniques such as this, these seventeen individuals became a group and, later, an ensemble.

Since the conditions imposed by life imprisonment are profoundly frustrating to the inmates, any experience that claims it can induce a move toward cohesiveness or solidarity will in fact be reality-tested by the inmates. Deprived of their liberty and worldly possessions, divested of personal autonomy, and compelled to associate with other deviants, prisoners become overwhelmed with anger, frustration, despair, and alienation. No experience can move them towards cohesiveness unless it has a deep integrity. The music program was clearly moving them in this direction, and rather quickly. If--as indeed it did--the music program had such power over aggressive and alienated prisoners in such a hostile environment, then there can be little doubt of its value and importance or of its potential in other environments.

In discussions that followed each daily session, any behavioral changes in the individual or the group as a whole were noted by the writers. From daily logs, profiles were developed for the group and for each participant. Patterns began to emerge, reasonably identifiable with each inmate. A study of these patterns and research into the psychological literature--in particular, the nonverbal domain--led to the discovery of *Theraplay*, a psychological intervention strategy based on deficits in human growth and behavior.[1] According to the author, Dr. Ann M. Jernberg, the basis for pathology, and, by implication, any inhibitors to growth, is found in a person's deficits in early SCIN experience. (SCIN is an acronym for Structuring, Challenging, Intruding, and Nurturing.) According to Jernberg, structuring is a need for definition, organization, and limitation. Challenging is the act of teasing and, occasionally, frustrating. Intruding is the process of exciting, stimulating, and surprising. And nurturing is indulging, reassuring, approving, and caring.

Diagnosing the SCIN deficits of an individual is one of the most important aspects of pretheraplay techniques. In the prison music program, the daily logs of observed behavior were the source for pretheraplay diagnosis. Using the Jernberg technique, modified to fit the circumstances, a SCIN profile--a graph of the individual's SCIN deficits and surplusses--took shape as a consequence of daily analysis of logged behavior. The process that emerged and the results observed were such that the teaching role increasingly took on a therapeutic orientation. Consequently, dividing lines between the roles of teacher and of therapist became obscured. The treatment was applied within the framework of group and private music lessons. It was discovered that if the psychological needs of a personality were to be met, they would be fulfilled in the nonverbal dimension of the music lessons or not at all.

The therapeutic functions inherent in the musical instruction were also clearly evidenced in the changing behavior within the group. Success in the mastery of even the simplest musical tasks was accompanied by an unexpected nonverbal group cohesiveness. This in turn gave rise to a sense of cooperation and mutual consideration quite foreign to the population of the institution.

From extended observations and analysis of the active nonverbal dimensions (individual and group instruction), certain precepts were generated.

First and foremost, the teacher must be in charge at all times. The teacher must also:

1. Be confident, highly capable, and have leadership qualities
2. Anticipate the student's resistant maneuvers and his own consequent actions before, *not after* they are set in motion
3. Be sensitive and responsive to cues given by students

---

[1]Ann M. Jernberg, *Theraplay* (San Francisco, California: Jossey-Bass, 1979).

4. Initiate rather than react to student participation
5. Insist on eye contact while talking
6. Place intensive and exclusive focus on the student
7. Recognize students' moods and failings and turn them away from unnecessary anxiety
8. Help the students come to terms with feelings
9. Keep the lessons spontaneous, flexible, and enjoyable
10. Keep each lesson optimistic and positive
11. Structure the lessons so that times, places, and persons are clearly defined
12. Offer some minimal challenges, frustration, and discomfort
13. Conduct each session without regard to personal feelings about the student
14. Focus on the present and the future
15. Focus on the student as he is
16. Maintain an insistent presence throughout the duration of the lesson

This list is not intended to be exclusive or complete. It only suggests some of the most important active, nonverbal factors that were found to be essential to the dual verbal and nonverbal teaching of music in the prison setting. Adherence to these precepts contributes to recognizable changes in behavior. They include:

1. A dramatic decrease in Discipline Reports recorded for members of the program
2. A decrease in negative proclivities
3. A willingness to become a member of a group with shared, nonmaterialistic objectives
4. An increased friendliness toward one another
5. Increased effort in the face of challenge
6. An increase in spontaneity and personal caring
7. A sense of group pride
8. A willingness to accept the advice of the instructor to pursue further educational opportunity
9. The ability to achieve peak experience
10. An increase in self-confidence, -esteem, and -satisfaction
11. A new pride in physical self-image as manifested in clothing and grooming

It is clear from the results of the six years of this program that voluntary participation in such a music program can contribute to such social and personal adjustment needs as conformity, experiencing group cohesiveness, discovering the uniqueness of one's role, and the need for cooperation. Participation may also be viewed as a dependable or potential advantage that is linked to the basic objectives of intervention. The results tend to indicate that a program in the prison setting, while not primarily rehabilitative in original intent, can accomplish substantial rehabilitative results. Exploration of the effectiveness of these methods applied in other settings might achieve similar results.

MAKING SCHOOL MUSIC PROGRAMS ACCESSIBLE
FOR THE HANDICAPPED

by

ROBERT H. KLOTMAN

This paper addresses music programs for the handicapped from the perspective of a music educator and administrator who, although not a specialist in the area, has had many years of experience with the problems inherent in mainstreaming. The paper will, therefore, deal essentially with suggestions or approaches that have been used in a variety of situations.

At Roosevelt Junior High School in Cleveland Heights, Ohio, where the writer was a music teacher from 1948 to 1956, there was a class of "exceptional" children who were identified as slow but "educable" learners. In addition to having a regularly scheduled general music class, several of the children in this group were learning to play formal instruments. There were three bands and three orchestras in the school-beginning, intermediate, and advanced. All children progressed from one performing group to the other as they developed technically and musically. Since all learners progress at different rates of speed, flexibility was essential. To help those children with learning disabilities make appropriate progress, the writer would rewrite parts so that even those who ordinarily could not develop beyond the most elementary stage were able to play even in the so-called advanced groups. It is important to remember that this was not a case of handing out contrived instruments but actually having an "exceptional" student play third trombone or fourth trumpet in a group going to music contests.

In altering the parts played by these children, notes were restricted to six notes on the scale. It was found that all of these children could function quite comfortably within this range. The rhythms were simplified so that while most of the performers might be playing rapid passages, others would be playing a sustained ostinato or a simple rhythmic background. To further assist these young people, other students at the same technical level were asked to share a desk with the "mainstreamed" child so that he or she could provide a model and assist that student during a performance. Incidentally, these helpers were young people who might be in an intermediate group, and by sharing a desk with an exceptional child in the advanced group, they were actually being given advanced opportunities and were delighted with the chance to assist. Everyone not only felt like a contributing member of the ensemble but also achieved a measure of personal satisfaction and self-esteem. The major obstacle to such an adjustment is merely the willingness on the part of the music teachers to rewrite the parts.

As a music administrator in Akron, Ohio and Detroit, Michigan, the writer was responsible for planning and organizing children's concerts in those communities. Although it was not until the 70s that the law required anyone receiving federal funds or support from any source to provide accessibility to all programs for handicapped children where appropriate, this program was already making efforts in the 60s to fulfill that responsibility. The Ohio program provided specially equipped seating for the hearing impaired at school concerts given by the Cleveland Orchestra. Their particular section had seats that were wired with hearing aids to assist those with limited hearing ability. In addition, signers were placed in strategic positions so that they could relay to the children the conductor's so-called appreciation portion of the program or his comments involving comprehension of the music. It should be noted that this group of children was seated in an inconspicuous area so that those in attendance at the concert were hardly aware of their presence. This was done to eliminate any self-conscious feelings that might occur. Special advanced printed materials, such as conductor's scripts, were forwarded to the teachers so that they could prepare these children beforehand.

Much can be done with the hearing impaired; the available technology has not yet begun to be used. Richard Hoke, a technology specialist at Gallaudet College, Washington, D.C., has described a specific instance of such use:

> Some deaf youngsters are even dancing without music at an elementary school on the Gallaudet campus, where a special dance floor is suspended over an air cushion. The result: a reverberating platform that vibrates to the music, allowing dancers to pick up the beat.[1]

As the article states, technology has provided a whole world of entertainment, and learning experiences are opening up for those of us who are educators. Music teachers need to become more aware and better informed as to what can be done with new developments to assist the arts in accommodating handicapped children.

In 1965-66, with money provided under the Elementary-Secondary Education Act, the Detroit, Michigan schools were able to sponsor a tour of the Mery-Go-Rounders, a New York-based

---

[1]Stanley Wellborn, "Deafness: America's 'Invisible' Handicap," *U.S. News and World Report,* 19 October 1981, p. 58.

children's ballet company. Arrangements were made for blind children to attend the program, while volunteers and teachers sat with them and described what was occurring on stage as they listened to the music. Anything said to describe the joy and pleasure expressed on these children's faces would be inadequate. Again, preprogram material was sent to the teachers so that the children could anticipate what would be occurring in the ballet. Furthermore, the Merry-Go-Rounders did a great deal of verbalizing so that the children were "visualizing" much of what was being performed on stage.

Placing program notes on cassettes is the next step. The advantage of this approach over braille is accessibility. Brief messages from a variety of sources, such as the concertmaster or the conductor, could be included. The advantage of cassettes is that copies can be made, and children may even take them home.

Children who are classified as exceptional or handicapped have the same needs for encouragement, love, respect, and feelings or self-esteem that all children do. Every child is unique, and the sensitive, exceptional educator will find ways to meet the needs of each child regardless of his or her special concerns. Music educators have a head start, for: "The use of the musical arts has long been recognized as a viable, effective teaching tool for the handicapped as well as a way of reaching youngsters who had otherwise been untouchable."[2]

The writer is of the opinion that goals and objectives in music education are meritorious for all children, whether they be normal or exceptional. In providing for handicapped children, there need only be adjustments and changes made to ensure that goals and demands are appropriate to the individual child's "exceptionality." Flexibility and creativity are the key guidelines. Musical demands should be so adjustable that they do not cause any child to be confronted with unnecessary failure. Music must not be another subject that dooms exceptional children to disappointment and heartbreak. It is imperative that "other children" be prepared before the "exceptional children" participate in activities with them.

Unfortunately, handicapped children always have and always will have their share of failure as a result of their inability to compete with the norms established in so many areas of the regular school curriculum. Music has so much to offer exceptional children

[2]Congressional Act, "Full Opportunity Goals," *Federal Register* 42, no. 163, 23 August 1977,

that when it comes to failure resulting from rigidity and inappropriate curricular standards, music education should stand out as the "exception."

IS LEFT-HANDEDNESS A HANDICAP FOR MUSICIANS?

by

IRVING B. PHILLIPS

Introduction

The purpose of this paper is: (a) to introduce the topic of handedness, (b) to outline and review the important research available on handedness with regard to musicians and musicianship, (c) to describe a recent study on handedness in a population of musicians and nonmusicians, (d) to describe the relationship between handedness and choice of musical instrument, (e) to describe a recent study that explored the relationship of handedness and teaching style in a sample population of student musicians, and (f) to explore the issue of left-handedness as a handicap for musicians.

Society is structured for the right-handed person and usually provides right-handed school desks, right-handed scissors, etc. In addition, there has been the custom of changing left-handed persons to right-handedness, and the enduring cultural bias against the left-hander since the dawn of recorded time. The Bible mentions a census that includes both right- and left-handed persons. The ancient Romans used "sinister" to describe the left-hander and also to describe those things associated with evil. Unfortunately, the bias continues to some extent today.

Left-Handedness as a Handicap

The controversy over the issue of handedness has persisted for centuries. Prior to this century, there was a definite bias against those who were left-handed. During our own century, there were those who perpetuated the myth that the left hand should not be used for any meaningful purpose. Schonberg (1967), for example, quotes Richard Strauss:

> The left hand has nothing to do with conducting. Its proper place is in the waistcoat pocket, from which it should emerge to restrain or to make some minor gesture--for which in any case a scarcely perceptible glance should suffice. (p. 237)

Is the left-hander handicapped with regard to music learning and performance? Is there anything related to music that the left-handed musician would find difficult because of handedness considerations? There is evidence that a normal population contains 13% left-handers (Spiegler & Yeni-Komishian, 1983). There is also evidence to suggest that the population of learning disabled students who are left-handed may be as high as 30%. Is this true for the population of musicians?

Is Left-Handedness a Handicap for Musicians?

There is a question as to whether or not researchers have investigated handedness in populations to determine if there is any difference with regard to handedness, musical ability, and proficiency considerations. Oldfield (1969) reported that there was no difference in handedness for musicians. The study showed that proportions of left-handed and right-handed musicians remained constant. The sample, however, consisted of an available college-level student and faculty population in England. Even though no differences were found, the results were not generalized to other segments of the musical population.

The Oldfield study began with the initial submission of 34 questions to a sample of college faculty and student musicians. This sample was composed of instrumentalists, pianists, vocalists, and a limited number of string players. Conducting was considered to be a musical instrument. On the basis of this sample, Oldfield concluded that there was no difference in handedness among musicians. The results of the study are questionable for two reasons: conducting was considered to be a musical instrument, and there was an inadequate sample of string players.

This first study by Oldfield has a redeeming factor: the development of the handedness inventory. An item analysis of each test question is contained in a later study by Oldfield, but not in this early study. Consequently, the test used for the earlier study was not validated. The 1971 short-form version of the test contains 10 test questions, while an early version contains 20. The shorter form of the test eliminated redundancies that were present on earlier tests. However, it was the first test that was used by Oldfield to draw conclusions concerning handedness in a sample population of musicians.

In a partial replication of the Oldfield study, Byrne (1974) expanded the study by including the issue of musical ability. Byrne used the short-form version of the Oldfield *Edinburgh Handedness Inventory* (Oldfield, 1971) on a sample larger than Oldfield's that contained both musicians and nonmusicians. Using two segments of the *Seashore Test* (timbre and tonal memory) and an IQ measure, Byrne found that there was no relationship among handedness, musical ability, and intelligence. The validity of Byrne's conclusions are in doubt because he did not identify the particular version of the *Seashore Test*. Since Byrne's study is dated 1974, it might have been more appropriate for him to choose a more contemporary test such as the Musical Aptitude Profile (MAP). Both Oldfield and Byrne had collected data on a sample population that reflected only a segment of the musical population. There was also the question of whether or not differences were to be found with regard to handedness in younger, nonprofessional student musicians.

There are several reasons why the Oldfield and Byrne studies were chosen for examination. First, both studies constitute a major portion of the literature with regard to handedness and music. Next, both studies are flawed by the same type of sampling error (the available college faculty and student sample). Further, the Oldfield study was the basis for the *Edinburgh Handedness Inventory*, which also appeared as the *Handedness Inventory Short Form*. This test has been widely used and has been discussed and compared to other handedness inventories (Varney & Benton, 1975; Crovitz & Zener, 1962; and Bryden, 1982). The *Edinburgh Handedness Inventory Short Form* is accompanied by an extensive item analysis. Such analyses are absent from other handedness tests.

The handedness test of Varney and Benton includes questions that solicit information regarding familial handedness; that is, the handedness of family members. Since this information is not requested on the *Edinburgh Handedness Inventory*, this researcher did seek that information when administering the test to subjects who participated in a study exploring the relationship of handedness and teaching style.

Musicians, Nonmusicians

A recent study by the writer (Phillips, 1985) involved samples of entire grades within a school district (4th, 7th, and 10th graders in the Canandaigua City School District in upstate New York), along with an entire college freshman class from the Eastman School of Music (a national population). The population included: beginning instrumentalists, singers, and a pianist. The skills levels encompassed three intervals, culminating with what is an almost professional sample of Eastman School freshmen.

Subjects were asked to complete the *Edinburgh Handedness Inventory Short Form*. In addition, they were requested to indicate if they were currently studying any musical instrument. The *Edinburgh* test asks the respondent to identify which hand is used for the following: writing, drawing, throwing, scissors, toothbrush, knife (without fork), spoon, broom (upper hand), striking a match (match), and opening a box (lid).

First, the population was examined with regard to handedness, and it was found to have no differences due to handedness. This indicated that the samples were representative of what had been predicted (about 11%).

Among Musicians

The next step was to evaluate the samples, (musicians and nonmusicians) in terms of handedness. A chi-square analysis of all groups indicated that handedness existed as a difference among the groups. However, when grades were analyzed separately, the issue of handedness was significant only with the fourth-grade group. There were significantly more right-handed fourth-grade musicians than that of left-handed fourth-grade musicians. An analysis of the data was also made by gender. Gender was not a factor.

Among Musicians by Instrument

Student respondents to the handedness inventory were asked to identify any instruments they were studying. Results of this analysis indicated that continuation on an instrument was not affected by handedness. The analysis grouped instruments in the following classifications: woodwinds, brass, strings, and other (including voice, piano, percussion, and harp). There was no significant difference within groups with regard to handedness.

Although musical instruments are played with both hands, there seems to be an unconscious bias toward the right-hander. Keyboard instruments are constructed with the higher notes on the right side of the midline and the lower notes on the left side of the midline. Why not the other way around? The technique for playing certain musical instruments involves an unequal use of the hands. Examples of this are: the trumpet, French horn, trombone, tuba, and the bowed string instruments. Certain musical instruments are played with either equal use of hands or unequal use of hands. For example, there is an equal use of hands when playing the piano, percussion, flute, oboe, clarinet, saxophone, and bassoon. There is an unequal use of hands when playing the trumpet, French horn, trombone, baritone horn, tuba, violin, viola, cello and bass.

Left-Handedness and the Acquisition
of Musical Performance Skills

The second phase of the study involved the teaching of a set of twelve modules on marimba to a group (eight) of right-handed subjects and a group (eight) of left-handed subjects. Each group was divided in half, and each half was taught with either a linear (sequential) method of presentation or a Gestalt (imitative) approach. Students were pretested and posttested with the *Watkins-Farnum Performance Scale*. Results of the difference scores between these tests indicated that handedness did not affect a subject's performance on this bimanual performance task. This suggests two things: (1) left-handers were not seen to be handicapped for this task. As reported in Brinkman and Kuypers (1972), both hemispheres of the brain are active even though fine motor tasks are lateralized for gross motor tasks; (2) handedness did not affect student performance significantly.

This suggests that here might be reason to suspect that even though the brain is lateralized for some stimuli, it may not be for complex tasks such as those involved with music performance. Psychologists such as Miran and Miran (1984) have recently called the entire problem of lateralization into question.

Conclusion and Summary

The data presented indicate that there is no significant difference between left-handed and right-handed musicians. Some of the data indicate that there may be certain advantages for either right-handers or left-handers during the acquisition of certain musical performance skills. This may take the form of increased skill in certain areas such as those associated with spatial or linear concepts. However, since both hands, both ears, and both eyes are required for the acquisition of these skills, it may be that the advantage for one skill may be the handicap for another skill. The net result is that left-handers and right-handers are essentially equal in the acquisition of musical performance tasks.

This equality was also evident in a limited study using two teaching methods. Even though there may have been advantages due to handedness, these advantages were not significant enough to support a hypothesis that handedness was a factor.

There was a difference in handedness for samples of musicians and nonmusicians at the fourth-grade level. Music instructors might now be inclined to consider students for instrumental study with slightly different critera than are presently being used.

Table 1
Handedness: Left to Right
by Grade Level
N=1154

Grade Level	Left	Right	Total
4	30	213	243
7A	31	286	317
7B	22	237	259
10	32	214	246
College Freshman	8	81	89
TOTALS	123	1031	1154

Table 2
Musicians and Non-Musicians
by Grade Level
N=1164

Grade Level	Musicians	Non-Musicians	Total
4	103	140	243
7A	80	242	322
7B	78	183	261
10	50	196	246
College Freshman	92	0	92
TOTALS	403	761	1164

Table 3
Raw Scores and Percentages:
Musicians and Non-Musicians
by Grade Level and Handedness
N=1154

Grade Level	Musicians				Non-Musicians				Total
	Left	%	Right	%	Left	%	Right	%	
4	7	7	96	93	23	17	117	83	243
7A	10	13	69	87	21	9	217	91	317
7B	11	15	66	85	13	8	169	92	259
10	5	10	45	90	27	14	169	86	246
College Freshman	8	9	81	91	0	0	0	0	89
TOTALS	41	10	357	90	84	15	672	85	1154

Table 4
Chi-Square Analysis
of Fourth Grade Musicians and Non-Musicians
by Handedness
N= 243

Handedness	Musician	Non-Musician	Total
Left	7	23	30
Right	96	117	213
Total	103	140	243

Chi-square$(1, \underline{N}=243)= 4.236$, $\underline{p}<.05$

Table 5
Chi-Square Analysis
of Seventh Grade (7A)
Musicians and Non-Musicians
by Handedness
N=317

Handedness	Musician	Non-Musician	Total
Left	10	21	31
Right	69	217	286
Total	79	238	317

Chi-square(1,$\underline{N}$=317)= .601, (not significant)

Table 6
Chi-Square Analysis
of Seventh Grade (7B)
Musicians and Non-Musicians
by Handedness
N=259

Handedness	Musician	Non-Musician	Total
Left	11	13	24
Right	66	169	235
Total	77	182	259

Chi-square(1,$\underline{N}$=259)= 2.488, (not significant)

Table 7
Chi-Square Analysis
of Tenth Grade Musicians and Non-Musicians
by Handedness
N=246

Handedness	Musician	Non-Musician	Total
Left	5	27	32
Right	45	169	214
Total	50	196	246

Chi-square$(1,\underline{N}=246)= .223$, (not significant)

Table 8
Chi-Square Analysis of
Musicians by Grade Level
and Handedness
N=398

	Handedness		
Grade Level	Left	Right	Total
4	7	96	103
7A	10	69	79
7B	11	66	77
10	5	45	50
College Freshman	8	81	89
TOTALS	41	357	398

Chi-square $(4,N=398)= 3.33823$, (not significant)

Table 9
Instrument Played
by Handedness:
Fourth Grade
N=101

Handedness	Instrument				
	Woodwind	Brass	String	Other	Total
Left	2	0	4	2	8
Right	30	10	24	29	93
Total	32	10	28	31	101

Chi-square(3,$\underline{N}$=101)= 2.62, (not significant⁾

Table 10
Instrument Played
by Handedness
Seventh Grade
N=153

Handedness	Instrument				
	Woodwind	Brass	String	Other	Total
Left	4	3	2	12	21
Right	30	18	14	70	132
Total	34	21	16	82	153

Chi-square(3,$\underline{N}$=153)= .1934, (not significant)

189

Table 11
Instrument Played
by Handedness
Tenth Grade
N=50

Handedness	Instrument				
	Woodwind	Brass	String	Other	Total
Left	0	2	0	2	4
Right	12	10	4	20	46
Total	12	12	4	22	50

Chi-square$(3,\underline{N}=50)= 2.65$, (not significant)

Table 12
Instrument Played
by Handedness
College Freshman
N=86

Handedness	Instrument				
	Woodwind	Brass	String	Other	Total
Left	3	0	3	2	8
Right	15	13	17	33	78
Total	18	13	20	35	86

Chi-square$(3,\underline{N}=86)= 3.794$, (not significant)

REFERENCES

Brinkman, J., & Kuypers, H. (1972). Splitbrain monkeys: Cerebral control of ipsilateral and contralateral arm, hand, and finger movements. *Science, 176,* 536-539.

Bryden, M. P. (1982). *Laterality: Functional asymmetry in the intact brain.* New York: Academic Press.

Byrne, B. (1974). Handedness and musical ability. *British Journal of Psychology, 65*(2), 279-281.

Crovitz, H. F., & Zener, K. (1962). A group test for assessing hand and eye dominance. *American Journal of Psychology, 75,* 271-276.

Miran, M., & Miran, E. (1984). Cerebral asymmetries: Neuropsychological measurement and theoretical issues. *Biological Psychology, 19,* 295-304.

Oldfield, R. C. (1969). Handedness in musicians. *British Journal of Psychology, 60*(1), 91-99.

Oldfield, R. C. (1971). The assessment and analysis of handedness: The Edinburgh Inventory. *Neuropsychologia, 9,* 97-113.

Phillips, I. B. (1985). Handedness and musical ability: An analysis of musicians and non-musicians and the relationship of handedness to a music teaching-learning paradigm (Doctoral dissertation, University of Rochester, Eastman School of Music, 1985).

Schonberg, H.C. (1967). *The great conductors.* New York: Simon & Schuster.

Spiegler, B. J., & Yeni-Komishian, G. H. (1983). Incidence of left-hand writing in a college population with reference to family patterns of hand preference. *Neuropsychologia, 21* (6), 651-659.

Varney, N. R., & Benton, A. L. (1975). Tactile perception of direction in relation to handedness and familial handedness. *Neuropsychologia, 13,* 449-454.

Watkins, J. G., & Farnum, S. (1954). *The Watkins-Farnum performance scale.* Winona, Minnesota: Hal Leonard Music.

THE DEPARTMENT OF REHABILITATION MEDICINE
NEW YORK UNIVERSITY MEDICAL CENTER
GOLDWATER MEMORIAL HOSPITAL

by

MATHEW H. M. LEE

The Department of Rehabilitation Medicine at Goldwater Memorial Hospital, New York City, composes a major segment of the clinical services provided under an affiliation agreement with the New York City Health and Hospitals Corporation. The hospital is rehabilitation oriented and provides care for long-term and disabled patients. While there is necessarily a statistical weighting in the direction of older patients, the patient population includes all ages with the general exception of children under fifteen. Even young children, however, are admitted under exceptional circumstances such as a need for extensive respiratory care. With the exception of respirator patients and amputees, out-patient services are not provided.

The Department has clinical responsibility for approximately 642 beds out of a total of 912 beds in the hospital. The Department of Medicine is directly responsible for the remainder of the beds, and the services of all other departments of the School of Medicine are available on a consultation basis.

Bed allocations in the Department are distributed as follows:

Acute Rehabilitation	192
Skilled Nursing Facility	
(extended care)	412
Respirator Service	38

In addition to clinical responsibility for its own beds, the Department of Rehabilitation Medicine also provides medical and paramedical services on a consultation basis for the entire hospital. A full range of paramedical services is included. The full-time medical staff of the Department of Rehabilitation Medicine consists of fourteen physicians. There is, in addition, a complement of six to seven resident physicians. Allocations for each of the paramedical disciplines are substantial.

A program for training and education for physicians and paramedical personnel is conducted. At the present time, in addition to intramural training, school affiliations are maintained with thirty colleges or schools from eleven universities in the various paramedical disciplines. Registered and practical nurses receive training in the service. An extensive program is conducted for training dental students in the problems of chronic disease. The entire senior class of the School of Dentistry of New York University is assigned to Goldwater on a rotating basis. In addition, there is a summer fellowship program for dental students.

A follow-up service for amputees is conducted in the community, as well as a respiratory follow-up service. Additional services that are component parts of the Department are: an orthotic service, a sizeable research section, and a cardiorespiratory and work physiology testing laboratory that serves the entire hospital. The Rehabilitation Laboratory is the only facility in the New York City area utilizing computerized equipment to assess the pulmonary status of the severely disabled neuromuscular patients. Additional exercise testing is now performed on the severely disabled in the work physiology unit.

Admissions to the Goldwater Rehabilitation Service are accepted from hospitals, physicians, social agencies, or any professional source. Patients are accepted who can profit from rehabilitation and whose needs are not purely custodial. Exclusions include: psychoses, malignancy, and tuberculosis. Among the services being offered by the Department of Rehabilitation Medicine are the following: physical therapy, speech and audiology, psychology, rehabilitation counseling, occupational therapy, public health nursing, social service, recreation, and pulmonary laboratory.

The Skilled Nursing Facility is an extended care facility in which a full range of clinical services is provided as needed. This facility was originally developed a decade ago around a philosophy that sought to provide care to long-term and disabled patients who no longer required care in the general hospital and who were unable to return to the community for a variety of reasons, including social, psychological, or medical ones. Since its inception, studies and experimentation have been carried on for the purpose of developing effective methods of appropriate care for this type of patient.

The Howard A. Rusk Respiratory Rehabilitation Service is unique in this part of the United States in terms of its specialization and facilities. Rehabilitation concepts are utilized in the service with the goal of improving breathing function. Originally established for the treatment of respiratory problems resulting from poliomyelitis, this service gradually added the treatment of chronic crippling respiratory conditions arising from other diagnoses. The rising number of emphysema patients and respiratory problems arising from other diagnoses has increased the demands on this service.

Many additional specialized programs currently being conducted in the Department of Rehabilitation Medicine include: biofeedback, geriatric group therapy, nonvocal communication, development of specialized prosthetic and orthotic equipment for severely disabled patients, cardiopulmonary testing, medical and psychological approaches to assessment and management of chronic pain, interdisciplinary approach to the treatment of decubitus ulcers, and a rehabilitation OPD clinic of discharged patients now living in the Roosevelt Island Community.

It is the philosophy of the Department that a high level of clinical care goes hand in hand with active professional involvement in teaching, clinical research, writing, lecturing, and the like. None of the activity overlooks the fact that the basic charge of the Department is to render clinical care. On the contrary, the scope of activity reflects the quality of the staff, the investment of personal time and commitment, and the vital way in which the clinical care is carried on. All of these factors are aimed at maintaining a high level of clinical care both now and in the future.

APPENDIX

Department of Rehabilitation Medicine
Administration Staff and Service Chiefs

Mathew H. M. Lee, M.D., Director

Augusta Alba, M.D., Deputy Director

Masayoshi Itoh, M.D., Associative Director, Skilled Nursing Facility; Administrative Physician, Skilled Nursing Facility

Herbert Zaretsky, Ph.D., Associate Director; Chief, Psychology Service

Marilyn Kream, B.B.A., Supervisor, Rehabilitation Administrative Services

Joan Adler, M.A., Chief, Rehabilitation Laboratories

Alice Eason, M.P.A., R.P.T., Chief, Physical Therapy Service

Gail Herring, M.S.W., Chief, Social Service

Patricia Kerman-Lerner, M.S., Chief, Speech Pathology and Audiology Service

Cynthia Links, M.A., Chief, Rehabilitation Counseling

Daniel Martins, C.O., Supervisor, Orthotics and Prosthetics

Hannah Shields, M.A., Chief, Therapeutic Recreation

Carmel Tuths, R.N., M.A., Chief, Public Health Nursing

Judith Wasserman, B.S., Chief, Occupational Therapy

LEARNING DISABILITIES IN POSTSECONDARY
MUSIC EDUCATION

by

GERALDINE WARD

Introduction

Over the past several years, many postsecondary music schools have been in a perplexing situation. For a variety of philosophical, economic, and demographic reasons, these schools have been giving serious consideration to applications of students who only a few years ago would have been rejected because of their high school records and test scores. In addition, it has become increasingly apparent that many students who choose to major in music are coming to higher education poorly prepared in the theoretical aspects of music as well as in other areas.

The Problem

Based on research (reported herein) at a major music school and the observations of other professional music educators over the past several years, evidence is growing and clearly suggests that a rather large percentage of this student population shows definite symptoms of various learning disabilities. Further, it suggests that in many cases the early emergence of music talent has disguised the problem; because of this talent, the music student has successfully avoided or been guided away from high school classes where the emphasis on reading and writing skills might have disclosed the learning difficulty.

Once in college, the problem is magnified for students and faculty alike. On the one hand, the rate of student attrition and the observed difficulty of those who choose to stay are both cause for concern. On the other hand, these problems have a direct effect on the faculty. Experienced and dedicated faculty members are finding that previously successful pedagogy just does not work with these students. The teachers feel that their present skills are not sufficient for the educational tasks they are expected to perform. At a time when student retention is a priority concern for every college, this combination of discouraged students and frustrated teachers has created a serious educational dilemma.

Experienced teachers with long-standing interest in the learning process have been puzzled by those students who, for no

196

apparent reason, have difficulty processing incoming information or recoding information for written or verbal communication. They are equally puzzled by the obviously talented students who seem to be working diligently but never seem to reach their potential. Research is showing that these students not only have difficulty in the liberal arts areas but also in learning music concepts in the classroom and in acquiring music performance skills in the studio.

The problems of accommodating students with special educational needs have received an increasing amount of attention in recent years at the local, regional, and national levels. However, **little if any consideration has been given to the effects of the prevalence of learning disabilities in college music teaching.**

The variety of the manifestations of learning disabilities, the nature of the music discipline itself, and the common institutional admissions procedures are working together to place the learning disabled in college music classrooms and studios.

Methods vary by which music majors are selected for college admission. They range from a virtual open admissions policy in a few institutions to an elaborate process that evaluates innate musicality as demonstrated through the performance medium, plus a review of all grades, test scores, and recommendations. Whatever combination of criteria is used, most admissions committees, encouraged by the National Association of Schools of Music, weight their decisions heavily on the actual performance skill of the candidate.[1] Thus, in many cases, the musically gifted student with a weak academic background is offered admission. This is not to imply that this policy is wrong or that it should be changed; it is offered as an explanation to those frustrated teachers and administrators and to those talented young people with slight to moderately severe learning disabilities who find themselves floundering in the college music curriculum.

Data, described later in the paper, along with anecdotal records of classroom experiences collected over the past four years, provide mounting evidence that the learning disabled student may encounter difficulty in any department of the music school. Because of their inadequate language-processing skills, these students are overwhelmed by even a minimum of assigned reading. Their reading is usually slow and arduous and is often accompanied by difficulty in determining the important information in a paragraph. Since they have limited ability to translate what they know into a coherent

---

[1]National Association of Schools of Music, *1985-1986 Handbook* (Reston, Virginia: National Association of Schools of Music, 1985), p. 43.

written form within the given time constraint, many find that answering examination questions in writing is an insurmountable task. Their answers often take the form of disorganized sentence fragments that may not indicate the level of their real understanding of the material. We all can remember the flutter of anxiety that accompanied the appearance of the blue test booklet. For these students, it is not a flutter; it is a hurricane of threatening proportion.

Although the learning disabled college music student may have acquired coping skills that allow him to muddle through a language-oriented course, there will have been few experiences in his educational past that have prepared him for functioning within the complex system of music notation that is required at the professional level. Therefore, the potential for failure is present in any music class.

Beyond descriptions in the professional literature of problems that learning disabled students have with the language symbol system, this research has led to a growing compendium of difficulties they may encounter with the music symbol system. The following are a few examples:

1. The inability to translate visual input into an auditory mode for sightsinging or silent scorereading

2. The inability to translate auditory input into a visual mode for taking melodic, rhythmic, or harmonic dictation

3. The inability to read a multi-part score because of figure/ground confusion

4. The inability to read vertical as well as horizontal lines of music

5. The inability to integrate, visually or auditorily, an open score into a composite of potential sounds

6. The difficulty associated with symbol reversals

7. The inability to read chord structures from bottom to top (as opposed to the direction of language reading)

Along with the visual and auditory perceptual deficiencies that are characteristic of these learners, there are often motor coordination problems. In conducting classes and secondary piano studios, the following difficulties are readily observed:

1. Deficiencies in fine motor control and/or coordination

2. The inability to integrate the visual input with the appropriate motor cue

3. The inability to coordinate cueing and interpretive gestures while maintaining a beat pattern in conducting

4. The inability to read simultaneous lines of music notation

5. The inability to maintain an awareness of the position of the various body parts in space, e.g., elbows, shoulders

6. The lack of clearly defined right- or left-handedness

7. The inability to cross the body midline in order to maintain pattern and the gesture accuracy in conducting

Finally, many learning disabled students demonstrate difficulties that seem to be based on three overriding problems: (1) deficiencies in skills of verbal communication, (2) deficiencies in organizational skills, and (3) defeating attitudes about themselves not only as learners but as worthwhile and capable individuals. These problems may result in the following behaviors:

1. An inability to speak in clear, well-organized sentences

2. The persistence of fragmentary verbalizations, often accompanied by unstructured and irrelevant arm movements and frequently followed by such phrases as "you know what I mean"

3. A persistent inability to organize time and study schedules. (Many of these students seem to live in a constant swirl of lost papers, forgotten appointments, and missed deadlines.)

4. An inability to organize and carry through a long-range plan. (A term paper is Mt. Everest to someone who cannot organize his life between 8:00 A.M. and 9:00 A.M.)

5. The tendency to cut classes rather than face the possibility of exposure or of another failure. (Students often report having cut class for which they **had prepared** out of fear that the pressure of the moment would cause an inability to per form. Many clearly understand that not attending classes is in itself defeating and are caught in a double bind.)

While this list of observed behaviors is long, it is by no means complete. And, of course, no single behavior taken by itself is enough to indicate a learning disability. However, when a student's record shows an emergent pattern of several of these behaviors, it is imperative that the pattern be recognized and evaluated.

Until the initiation of this study, recognition of patterns was difficult because of the structure of the music school faculty. There was little opportunity for any single faculty member to have ready access to information about the student's specific difficulties or successes in other studios or departments.

The Study

In fall 1981, a longitudinal study that now includes students from four successive incoming classes at Westminster Choir College (a professional school of music in Princeton, New Jersey) was initiated. The subjects, now numbering 251, are all native born, first-time college students. Transfer students and international students are not included. Information has been collected that covers the following areas: sex, performing medium, scores from the Scholastic Aptitude Tests, the Test of Standard Written English, the Basic Musicianship Evaluation (a college-prepared evaluation of rhythmic responses and pitch discrimination), the Aliferis Test (a validated music aptitude test), and an ongoing compilation of cumulative grade point averages and/or withdrawal information (i.e., in satisfactory or unsatisfactory academic standing).

Of these students, 240 (96%) have completed a self-evaluation survey that includes questions pertaining to: motor skills; aural, visual, and tactile perception; reading and study habits; and sequencing and organizational skills. This survey is given during freshman orientation week, before attendance at college classes or lessons. In addition, the *QNST: Quick Neurological Screening Test,* revised edition, has been administered individually to 106 (42%) of the subjects.[2]

These data, along with anecdotal information from faculty members, have been used in an attempt to identify those students in the study who seem to be at high risk of failure. Since the first group of students in the study have not yet finished their eighth

---

[2]M. Mutti, H. M. Sterling, and N. V. Spalding, *QNST: Quick Neurological Screening Test,* rev. ed. (Novato, California: Academic Therapy Publications, 1978).

semester, it is impossible to give hard data concerning final cumulative grade point averages and persistence to graduation. However, clear trends are becoming apparent.

Discussion of Preliminary Data

Course work involving those skills identified earlier is indeed the most common stumbling block to academic success. This is reflected in current cumulative grade point averages and in records of withdrawal and/or dismissal.

Of those students (N=138) who have been followed through five full semesters, thirty-four (24.6%) have left school in **unsatisfactory** academic standing. Twenty of these thirty-four students have been given the *QNST: Quick Neurological Screening Test* before leaving. The median score (21.850) of that group is appreciably higher (denoting greater suspicion of neurological difficulties) than the median score (14.364) of the fifty-five students who remain in school in good standing and who were similarly tested. Whether these differences will continue to obtain, as testing of students enrolled in later years continues and data are added, remains to be seen. It does appear to be significant enough to encourage further work.

The self-evaluation, as it was designed for this study, appears now to have less significance. While some of the correlations with the *QNST* scores have been encouraging, much more work needs to be done on individual items in the questionnaire. There is also the problem of timing of the administration of this survey. While freshman orientation week is a time when large groups can be organized for the task, it may not be the optimum time for thoughtful self-evaluation. The potential difficulties are many: some students may be psychologically ten feet tall, others may be wrestling with apprehension and self-doubt, and still others (incredulous about the reality of having been admitted to a professional music school) are loathe to admit to any previous difficulties.

Concurrent Academic Support

Shortly after the study began, a team of interested faculty members, all of whom teach some freshman courses, was formed for the purpose of creating a forum in which common classroom problems could be discussed and successful strategies shared. Since that time, a group of fifteen to eighteen of these high-risk students has been followed on a weekly basis. In addition to this special faculty attention, peer tutoring is started early with special training for the tutors preceding their work with the students. The list changes as students who seem to be making satisfactory progress are replaced by those needing faculty attention. Some of these high-risk students, at our suggestion, have sought testing and remediation off campus; others who could not afford these services have been helped only in our limited capacity on campus.

Several students are still enrolled who surely would have left school had they not had this attention. Unfortunately, there are others whose musical potential never came to fruition, in large part because the special services needed for academic success could not be provided.

More recently, this team has planned and presented two Faculty Effectiveness Seminars that were highly successful, although faculty attendance was voluntary. Faculty and administration interest in this project is high and their support is enthusiastic.

Obviously, the work has just begun. The difficulty of obtaining funding to expand the project is enormous; many agencies understand the problem but cannot seem to justify the allocation of funds for such a small and select segment of the total college population. Nevertheless, the search for funds will continue, and the work with these students will persist.

REFERENCES

Mutti, M.; Sterling, H. M.; and Spalding, N. V. *QNST: Quick Neurological Screening Test.* Rev. ed. Novato, California: Academic Therapy Publications, 1978.

National Association of Schools of Music. *1985-1986 Handbook.* Reston, Virginia: National Association of Schools of Music, 1985.